Dyslipidemia

Edited by Samy I. McFarlane

Published in London, United Kingdom

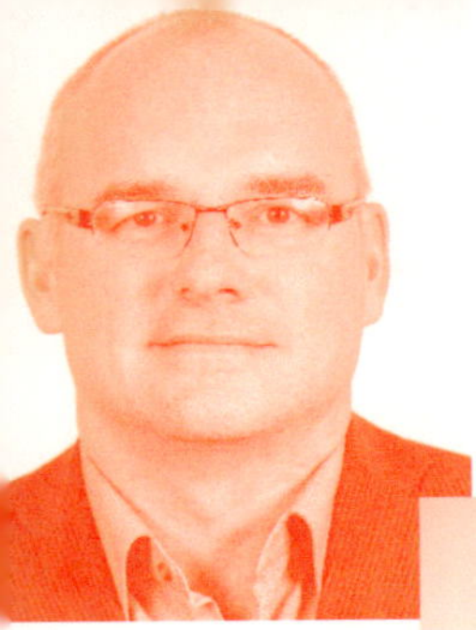
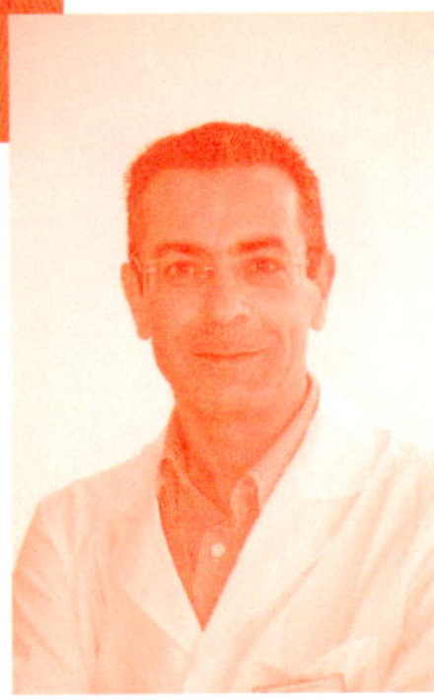
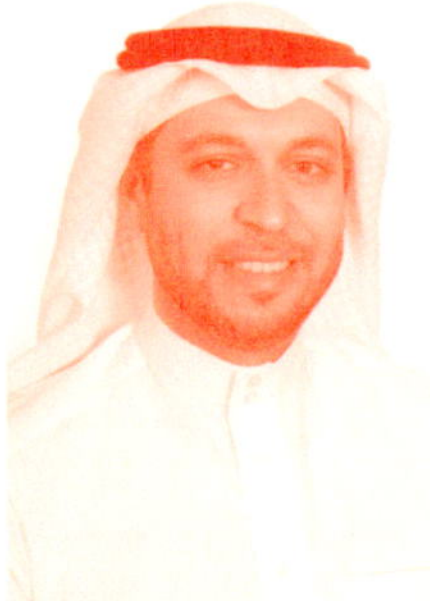
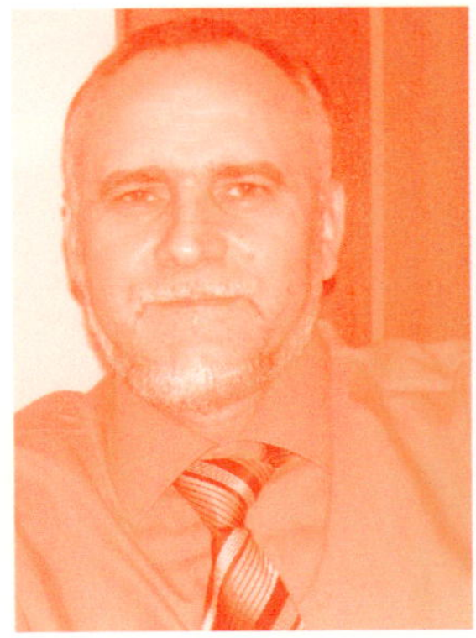
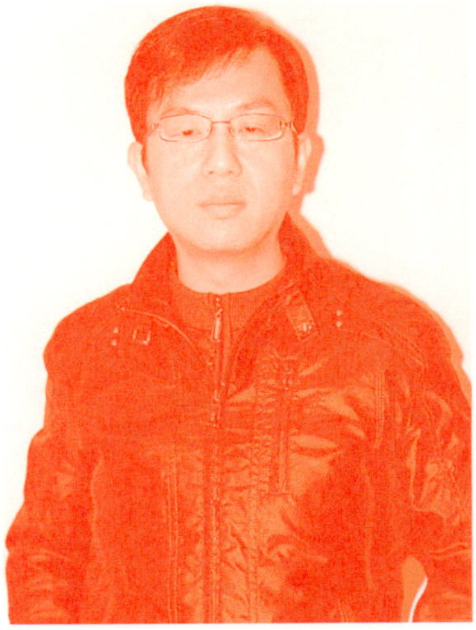
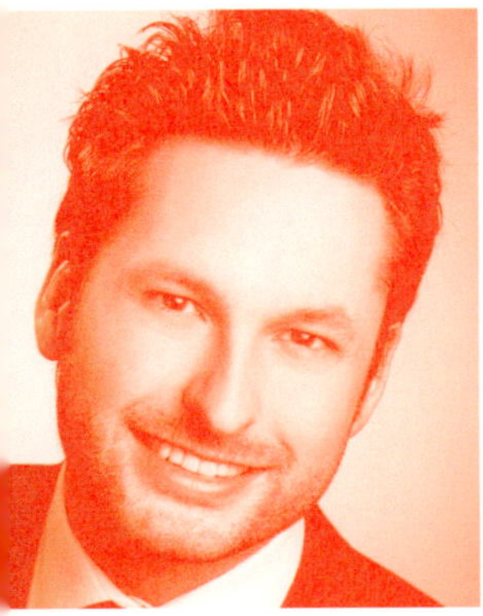
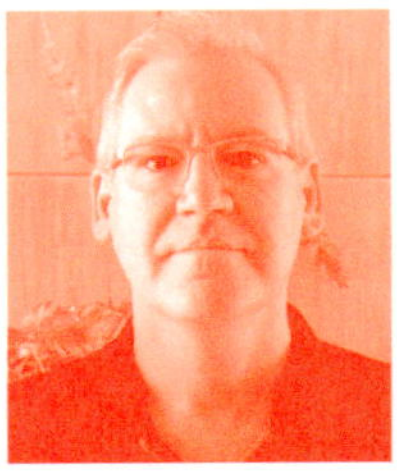

IntechOpen

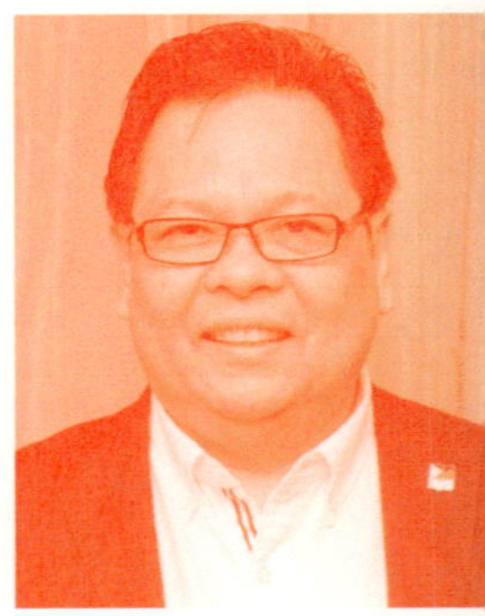
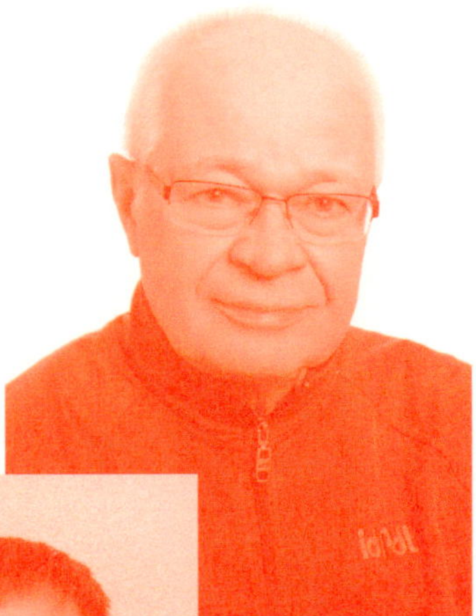
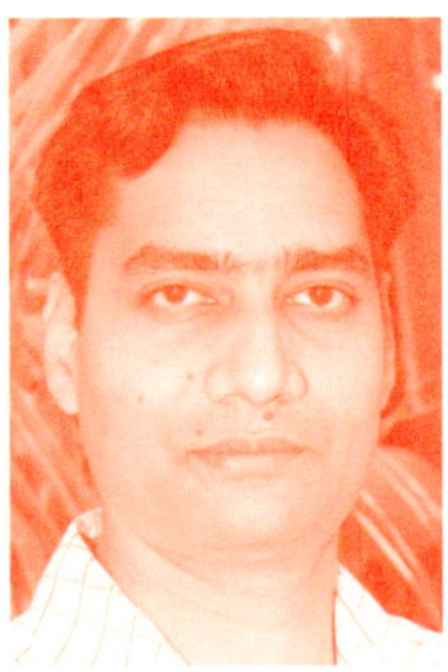
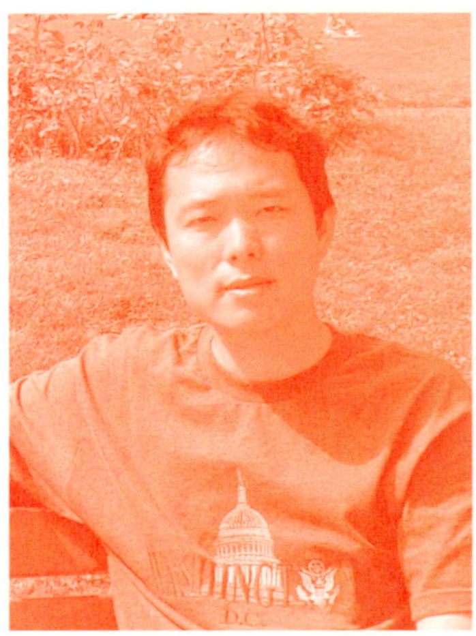
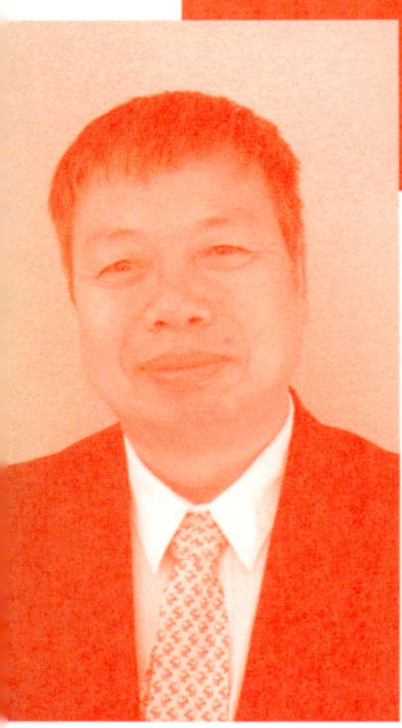
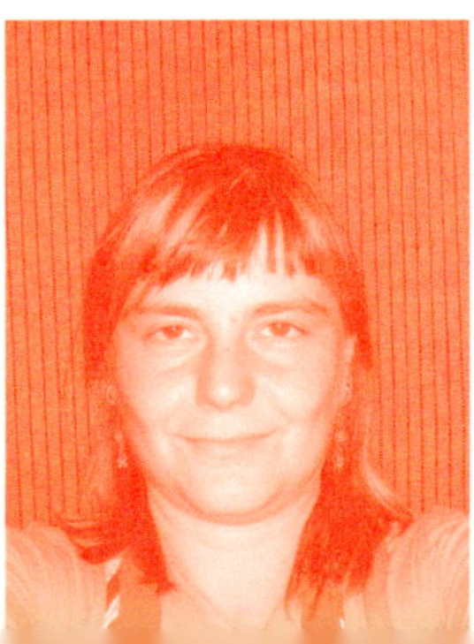

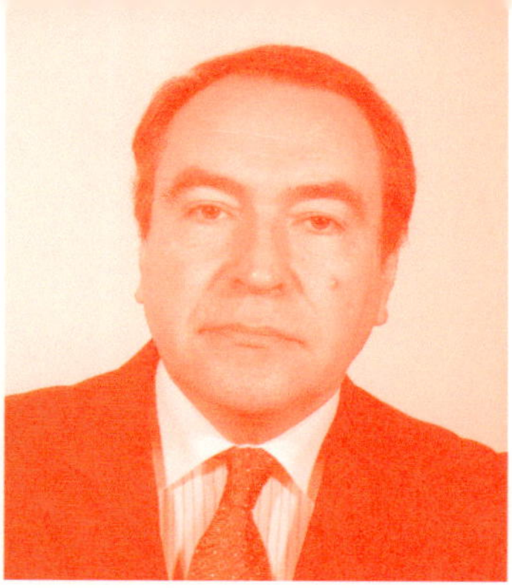
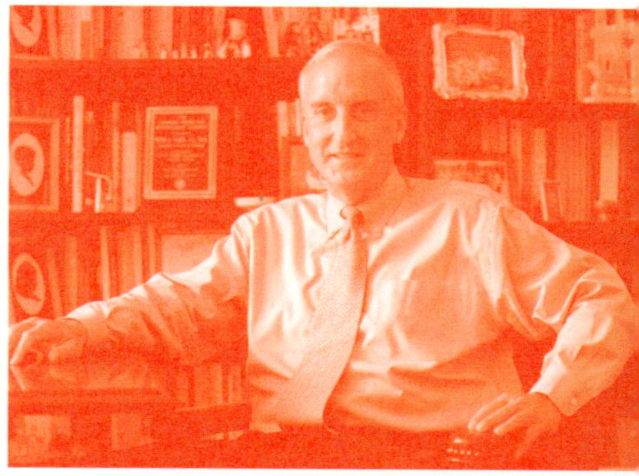
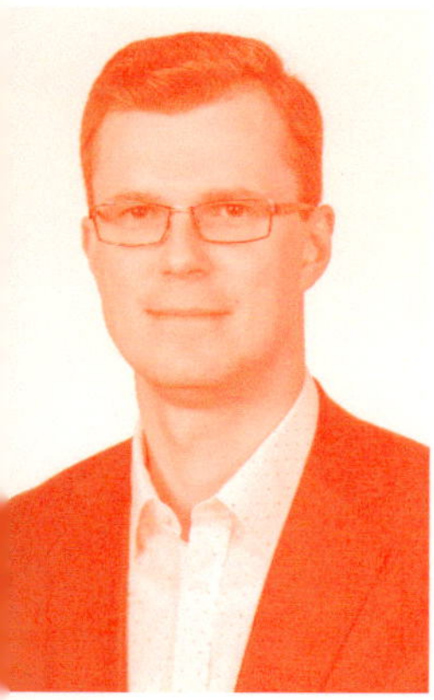
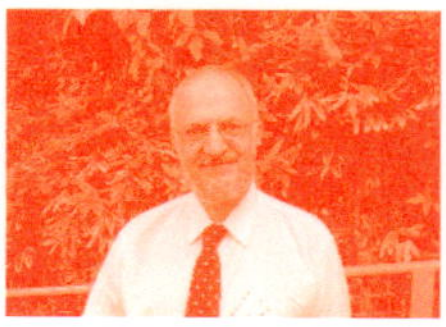
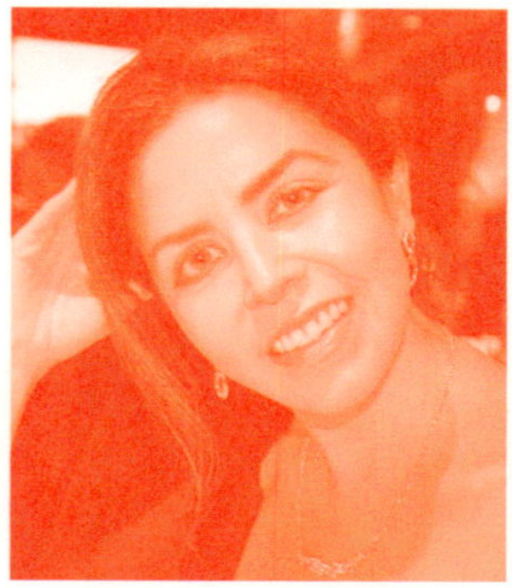

Supporting open minds since 2005

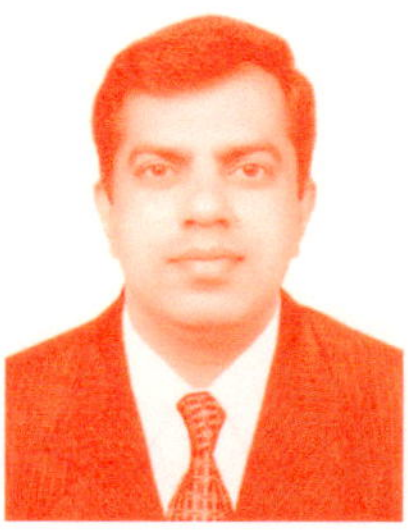
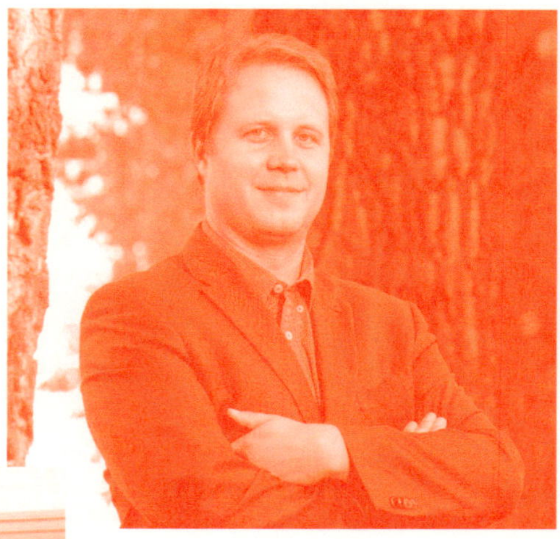
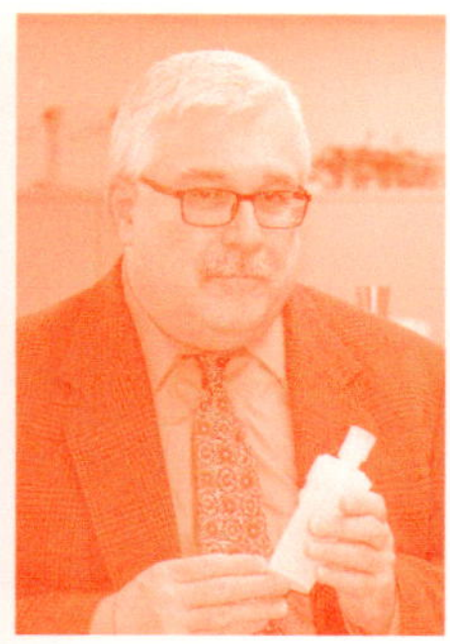
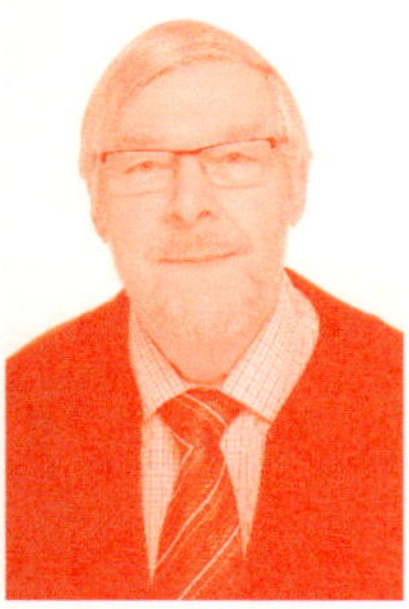
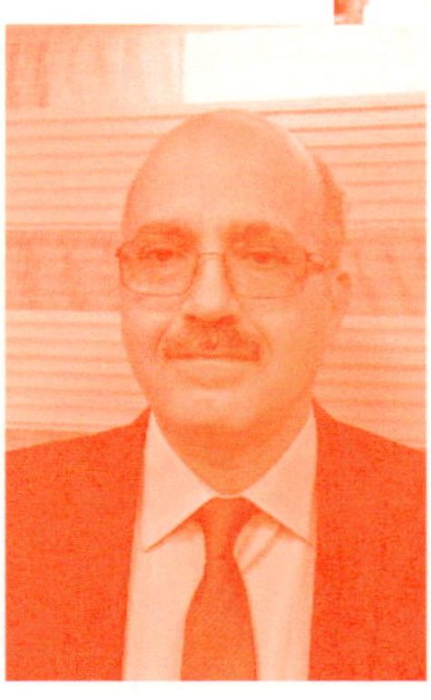
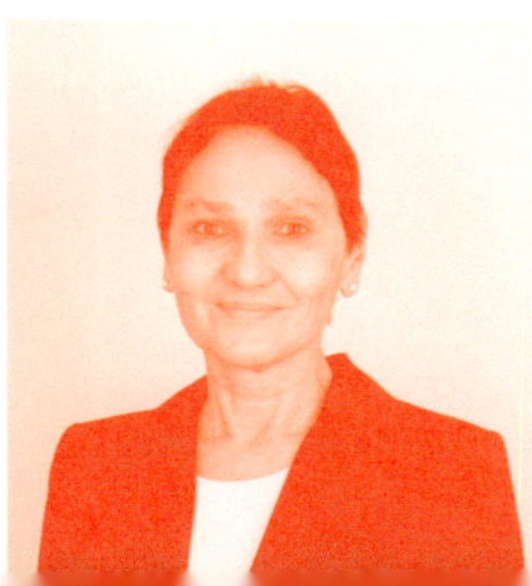
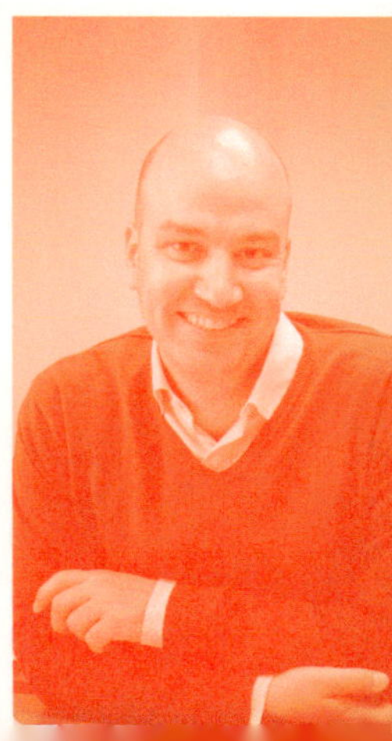

Dyslipidemia
http://dx.doi.org/10.5772/intechopen.76825
Edited by Samy I. McFarlane

Contributors
Joseph M. Keenan, Songkwan Silaruks, Charn Sriratanasathavorn, Petch Rawdaree, Rapeephon Kunjara-Na-Ayudhaya, Bandit Thinkhamrop, Piyamitr Sritara, Abdullah Glil Alkushi, Amarpali Brar, Clinton D. Brown, Moro O. Salifu, Jeans M. Santana, Samy I. McFarlane, Denis Yusupov, Angelina Zhyvotovska, Amgad N. Makaryus, Perry Wengrofsky, Justin Lee, Deborah R. Gustafson, Olta Tafaj Reddy, Leilani B. Mercado-Asis, Neil Francis Amba

First published in London, United Kingdom, 2019 by IntechOpen
IntechOpen is the global imprint of INTECHOPEN LIMITED, registered in England and Wales, registration number: 11086078, 7th floor, 10 Lower Thames Street, London, EC3R 6AF, United Kingdom
Printed in Croatia

British Library Cataloguing-in-Publication Data
A catalogue record for this book is available from the British Library

Additional hard and PDF copies can be obtained from orders@intechopen.com

Dyslipidemia
Edited by Samy I. McFarlane
p. cm.
Print ISBN 978-1-83968-003-8
Online ISBN 978-1-83968-004-5
eBook (PDF) ISBN 978-1-83968-005-2

For EU product safety concerns:
IN TECH d.o.o., Prolaz Marije Krucifikse Kozulić 3, 51000 Rijeka, Croatia, info@intechopen.com or visit our website at intechopen.com.

Meet the editor

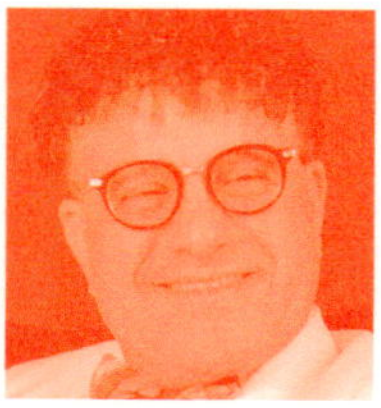

Dr. Samy I. McFarlane, MD, MPH, MBA, FACP is a distinguished teaching professor of Medicine and Endocrinology and an Associate Dean at the College of Medicine, State University of New York-Downstate Health Science University, USA.

He has extensive experience in clinical and translational research and has led the largest center in North America in the landmark diabetes prevention trial, the DREAM trial. He has edited several books and authored over 300 publications on diabetes, hypertension, dyslipidemia, cardiovascular disease, and related areas. His work has been among the most read articles with over 10,000 citations in major medical journals. He is the Founding Editor-In-Chief for the International Journal of Clinical Research and Trials and has served as the Editor-In-Chief for several other journals. He is a nationally and internationally recognized scholar who served as a member at the National Institute of Health-NIDDK committee (two terms) and as a chair of the NIH-NIDDK U01 review committee (twice). He has received multiple recognitions including Certificate of Special Congressional Recognition and he also served as District President for the American College of Physicians. He is also a well-recognized mentor with some of his trainees serving in leadership positions at the NIH and other major institutions.

Contents

Preface XI

Section 1
Introduction to Lipid Metabolism and the Role of Dyslipidemia in Atherogenesis 1

Chapter 1 3
Introductory Chapter: Overview of Lipoprotein Metabolism
by Angelina Zhyvotovska, Denis Yusupov and Samy I. McFarlane

Chapter 2 11
Dyslipidemia and Its Role in the Pathogenesis of Atherosclerotic Cardiovascular Disease: Implications for Evaluation and Targets for Treatment of Dyslipidemia Based on Recent Guidelines
by Perry Wengrofsky, Justin Lee and Amgad N. Makaryus

Section 2
Dyslipidemia in Special Populations 43

Chapter 3 45
Dyslipidemia in Special Populations, the Elderly, Women, HIV, Chronic Kidney Disease and ESRD, and Minority Groups
by Amarpali Brar, Jeans M. Santana, Moro O. Salifu and Clinton D. Brown

Chapter 4 71
Prevalence of Dyslipidemia and Goal Attainment with Lipid-Lowering Therapy: Insights from Thai Multicenter Study and Overview of the Major Guidelines
by Songkwan Silaruks, Charn Sriratanasathavorn, Petch Rawdaree, Rapeephon Kunjara-Na-Ayudhaya, Bandit Thinkhamrop and Piyamitr Sritara

Chapter 5 85
Postprandial Lipemia as Cardiovascular Disease Risk Factor
by Neil Francis Amba and Leilani B. Mercado-Asis

Section 3
Special Topics in the Management of Dyslipidemia 97

Chapter 6 99
Alternative Natural Management of Dyslipidemia
by Abdullah Glil Alkushi

Chapter 7 115
The Role of Niacin in the Management of Dyslipidemia
by Joseph M. Keenan

Chapter 8 129
Novel Therapies for Dyslipidemia
by Olta Tafaj Reddy

Section 4
Adiposity and Non-Tradional Lipid Biomarkers, a Look into the Future 143

Chapter 9 145
Adipose Tissue Complexities in Dyslipidemias
by Deborah R. Gustafson

Foreword

I am pleased to provide a preface for this comprehensive book on dyslipidemia edited by my mentee Professor Samy I. McFarlane. This book contains chapters that approach the science of lipid metabolism and the treatment of dyslipidemia from an international standpoint and in a wide variety of population groups. Several chapters deal with the etiology and treatment of dyslipidemia in high-risk populations such as those with HIV and patients with chronic kidney disease. Material in these chapters includes treatment goals in special populations and approaches to attain these goals. These special populations include Asian Indians, African Americans, and Hispanics, who are generally at a higher risk for dyslipidemia. Other chapters discuss the pathogenesis and treatment of dyslipidemia in these high-risk populations. This book also includes chapters that comprehensively discuss non-pharmacological, hygienic, and unconventional approaches to treating dyslipidemia in various populations. Included also are comprehensive discussions of the unique metabolism and responses to statin therapy in various groups, and the potential genetic factors underpinning these different responses to HMG-CoA Reductase inhibitors. This book presents unique approaches to the problem of dyslipidemia and this makes this book different from prior publications on this topic.

James R. Sowers, MD, FAHA
Director of Diabetes and Cardiovascular Research Center
University of Missouri

Preface

Dyslipidemia is a major risk factor for cardiovascular disease that is potentially modifiable and includes a heterogenous group of disorders commonly encountered in clinical practice. While several volumes addressing dyslipidemia had been previously published, this book presents a unique overview and sheds light on several topics that have not been sufficiently addressed in the literature. In this book, we assembled a group of nationally and internationally recognized scholars in their fields to share their experience and knowledge with the readers. We also provided an introductory chapter that deciphers the highly complex lipid metabolic pathways. The book highlights the pathogenesis of atherosclerosis with a focus on the role of dyslipidemia in cardiovascular disease, thus providing a rationale to treatment targets and practice guidelines. Also, unique to this book is the discussion of lipid disorders from an international perspective, addressing high-risk populations including ethnic groups such as Indians, Asians, Hispanics, and African Americans as well as those with certain disorders that heighten their cardiovascular risk such as HIV patients, chronic kidney disease, and end stage renal disease populations. Special focus on dyslipidemia in women and the elderly is also addressed. This non-traditional volume addresses non-traditional approaches to dyslipidemia including plant products such as gum residue and red yeast rice among many food supplements commonly used around the world in highly populated nations including India and China. Furthermore, a fresh look at some of the largely abandoned pharmacologic agents such as niacin and its utility in dyslipidemia management is presented by a world expert, providing new perspective on the subject. This, in addition to discussion on postprandial dyslipidemia, is a risk factor that is often overlooked in the evaluation and management of cardiovascular disease.

Finally, an updated review on the role of PCSK9 as a modern therapeutic agent is provided, together with a chapter on the emerging role of brown adipose tissue in dyslipidemia and cardiovascular risk. This is presented by a world expert on fat metabolism who also provides future insights into this highly active area of investigation. We believe that this book, *Dyslipidemia*, provides a basic understanding as well as advanced knowledge into lipid metabolism. This book should be useful to the student, researcher, as well as busy practitioner as it highlights cutting edge information and novel therapeutic approaches to dyslipidemia.

Samy I. McFarlane MD, MPH, MBA
State University of New York,
Downstate Medical Center,
United States

Section 1

Introduction to Lipid Metabolism and the Role of Dyslipidemia in Atherogenesis

Chapter 1

Introductory Chapter: Overview of Lipoprotein Metabolism

Angelina Zhyvotovska, Denis Yusupov and Samy I. McFarlane

1. Introduction into lipids

Dyslipidemia is a major cardiovascular disease (CVD) risk factor that is frequently encountered in clinical practice, affecting one in three adults (over 30% of adult population) in the United States alone [1, 2]. It is generally associated with other CVD risk factors including insulin resistance/diabetes, hypertension, and central obesity. With the publication of the landmark observational study, the Framingham Heart Study, the predictive relationship between hypercholesterolemia and coronary heart disease (CHD) was established, where adults with total cholesterol (TC) of >300 mg/dl were 5 times more likely to have CHD, compared with those of TC of <200 mg/dl [3]. These findings were further supported by data from another landmark study, the Multiple Risk Factor Intervention Trial (MRFIT) that clearly demonstrated a graded and strongly positive correlation between TC levels and CHD mortality [4]. Subsequently, multiple trials using various lipid-lowering agents clearly established CVD benefits from lipid lowering. For example, the Lipid Research Clinics Coronary Primary Prevention Trial (LRC-CPPT), using cholestyramine, a bile acid sequestrant, demonstrated that 1% reduction in TC led to 2–3% reduction in CHD risk [5]. Similarly, using gemfibrozil, a fibric acid derivative, in the Helsinki Heart Study, a 5-year primary prevention trial, there was 34% risk reduction in myocardial infarction and sudden cardiac death in the treatment group, compared to placebo [6]. With the advent of statins, numerous clinical trials have shown CVD benefits with cholesterol-lowering therapy that are above and beyond just lowering lipid levels [7]. These findings collectively reinforced the negative connotation associated with lipids in general, despite the vital roles lipids play in various metabolic processes such as the bi-lipid layer cell membrane, the formation of steroid hormones, and bile. In this introductory chapter to our book that addresses topical issues of dyslipidemia, we provide an introduction we believe will be useful to a wide range of audiences including students, researchers, and clinical providers with a simplified overview of the structure, classification, and metabolism of lipids. This chapter will serve as a quick and illustrated reference to the reader of this book, Dyslipidemia, thus facilitating the understanding of the other book chapters.

2. Classification of lipids

There are three types of lipids:
Simple lipids such as oil and waxes.
Complex lipids such as phospholipids, glycolipids, and lipoproteins.
Derived lipids such as steroid hormones and lipid-soluble vitamins.

3. Saturated and unsaturated fatty acids

Saturated fatty acids are those containing no double bonds such as acetic (CH_3—COOH) and palmitic acid (**Figure 1**).

Unsaturated fatty acids contain one or more double bonds and are divided into three categories: **Monounsaturated** (one double bond), **polyunsaturated** (two or more double bonds), and **eicosanoids** (derived from 20 carbons = eicosa) that include **prostaglandins**, **thromboxanes**, and **leukotrienes.**

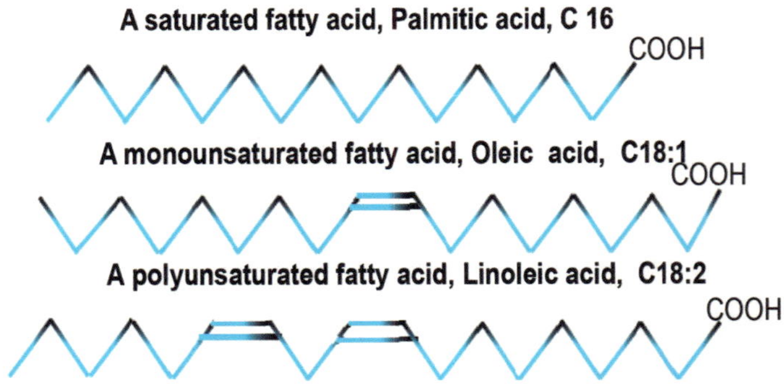

Figure 1.
Saturated and unsaturated fatty acids.

4. Cis and trans bonds

Cis and trans bonds are isomers of fatty acids (**Figure 2**); nearly, all naturally occurring bonds are in cis configuration. Trans fatty acids are the results of partial hydrogenation, a process that is used to create solidified products such as margarine. Trans fatty acids are proinflammatory, increase LDL and decrease HDL-cholesterol, and increase risk for obesity, diabetes, and CVD. These deleterious effects of trans fats prompted the FDA to ban the production of partially hydrogenated oils in June 2018. **Figure 2** illustrates how trans fats can stack neatly, one on top of the other, to create dense solid fats.

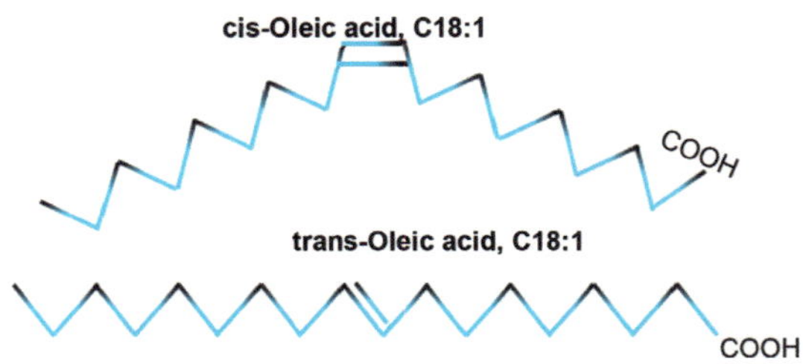

Figure 2.
Cis- and trans-oleic acid.

5. Overview of lipoprotein structure, function, and metabolism

Lipids are insoluble in water and are transported in the plasma (or extracellular fluids) by lipoproteins. These lipoproteins have, in their basic structure, a lipid core to be transported (triacylglycerols (TAG), phospholipids, and cholesterol esters). A hydrophilic layer in which apolipoproteins are embedded thus provides structural stability as well as identity for each type of the lipoprotein.

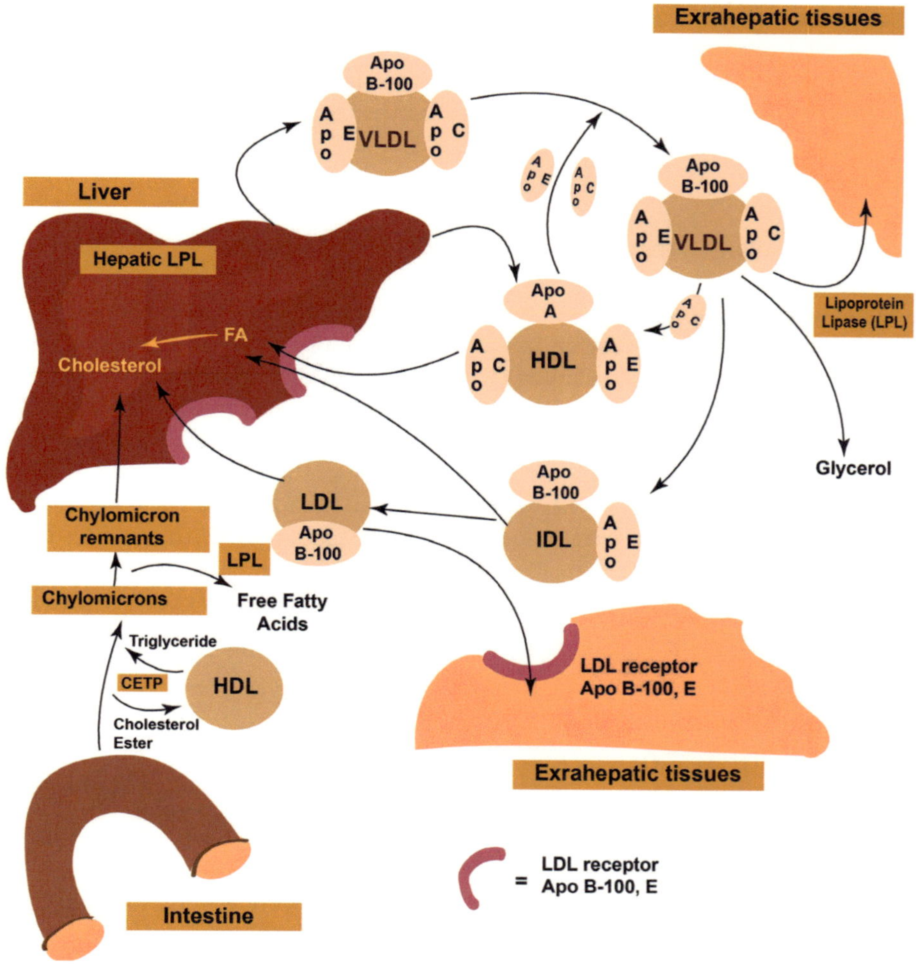

Figure 3.
Lipid transport and storage.

There are five major types of lipoprotein (**Figure 3**), classified based on their density (hence their size) from ultra-low-density lipoprotein (ULDL = chylomicrons) to very-low-density lipoprotein (VLDL), intermediate-density lipoproteins (IDL), and high-density lipoproteins (HDL). Chylomicrons (CM) are the largest in diameter with the lowest density and the highest TAG content.

Lipoprotein lipase is an enzyme that cleaves VLDLs and TAGs. TAGs are cleaved into free fatty acids and glycerol. Fatty acids eventually undergo **beta-oxidation**, and their energy is used by the heart and skeletal muscles. In the blood, free fatty acids are bound to albumin.

6. Exogenous (intestinal) lipid transport pathway

CM, formed in the intestinal epithelial cells (enterocytes), are the lipoproteins involved in the transport of exogenous (dietary) lipids from the intestine to the lymphatic system into the circulation through the exogenous lipid metabolism pathway (**Figure 3**). These CM contain cholesterol esters (CE) and TAG, formed by re-esterification of FFA, and are carried to the peripheral tissues including muscles and adipose tissues. By the action of activated LPL, FFA are released and undergo beta-oxidation to be used as energy source or stored as fat in the adipose tissues.

CM also, through the action of cholesterol ester transfer protein (CETP), acquire CE from HDL in exchange of TAG. Furthermore, CM in the lymphatic system exchange apo A-I and apo A-II for apo C and E from HDL. Apo C is required for the activation of the LPL, and apo E is required for the recognition of the CM remnants by the liver's receptors (**Figure 3**).

7. Endogenous lipid transport pathway

TAG and cholesterol from CM catabolism (remnants) are endogenously produced in the liver and are secreted in VLDL that contains apo B-100 (**Figure 3**). Similar to the process described above with CM, apo C and apo E are acquired from HDL where apo C activates LPL that catalyzes the hydrolysis of TG in VLDL producing FFA that are taken up by the muscles for energy production or stored in the adipose tissues. And again, as with CM, through the action of CETP, VLDL exchange cholesterol for TAG with HDL resulting in the formation of IDL which can be taken up by the liver via the apo E/remnant receptor or further reduced by hepatic lipase into LDL.

LDL contains only one apoprotein (B-100) and is taken up by the liver through LDL receptors with approximately one-third utilized by peripheral cells for membrane formation and steroidogenesis.

8. Reverse cholesterol transport pathway

This process involves the mobilization of cholesterol from the plasma membranes of cells along the arterial walls and the delivery of the cholesterol to the liver in the form of cholesterol esters (CE), thus reducing cholesterol levels in the periphery and thereby reducing inflammation as well as atherosclerosis.

In the macrophages of the vessel wall, CEs are hydrolyzed via cholesterol ester hydrolase (CEH), thereby releasing free cholesterol. This free cholesterol is transported outside the macrophages via adenosine triphosphate-binding cassette transporter A1 (ABCA1) to apolipoprotein A1, forming nascent pre-β HDL. The free cholesterol is then esterified into CEs via lecithin-cholesterol acyltransferase (LCAT), and the nascent pre-β-HDL then becomes mature α-HDL which converts into mature α-HDL subtypes, α-HDL2 and α-HDL3. This process occurs in the vessel walls as well as in the plasma and is mediated by LCAT as well as hepatic lipase (HL) and endothelial lipase (EL). Mature α-HDL2 and α-HDL3 continue to acquire free cholesterol delivered from inside the cells via ABCG1, therefore increasing the amount of cholesterol carried to the liver via the CE-rich α-HDL via either direct or indirect pathways (**Figure 4**).

In the direct hepatic cholesterol uptake pathway, CE-rich α-HDL binds to scavenger receptor B1 (SR B1) that recognizes Apo A1, and CEs are taken by hepatocytes and excreted in bile. In the indirect hepatic cholesterol uptake pathway, CE-rich α-HDL exchanges CE for TAG from the TAG-rich LAD and VLDL particles, a process that is facilitated by CETP, thereby forming a TAG-rich HDL and CE-rich LDL and VLDL. CEs are then taken by hepatocytes via LDL receptors, catabolized, and also excreted in the bile, as with the direct pathway.

The processes described above are well regulated in healthy states and are quite abnormal in dyslipidemia, leading to excess CVD as well as other disorders such as nonalcoholic fatty liver disease (NAFLD), among others.

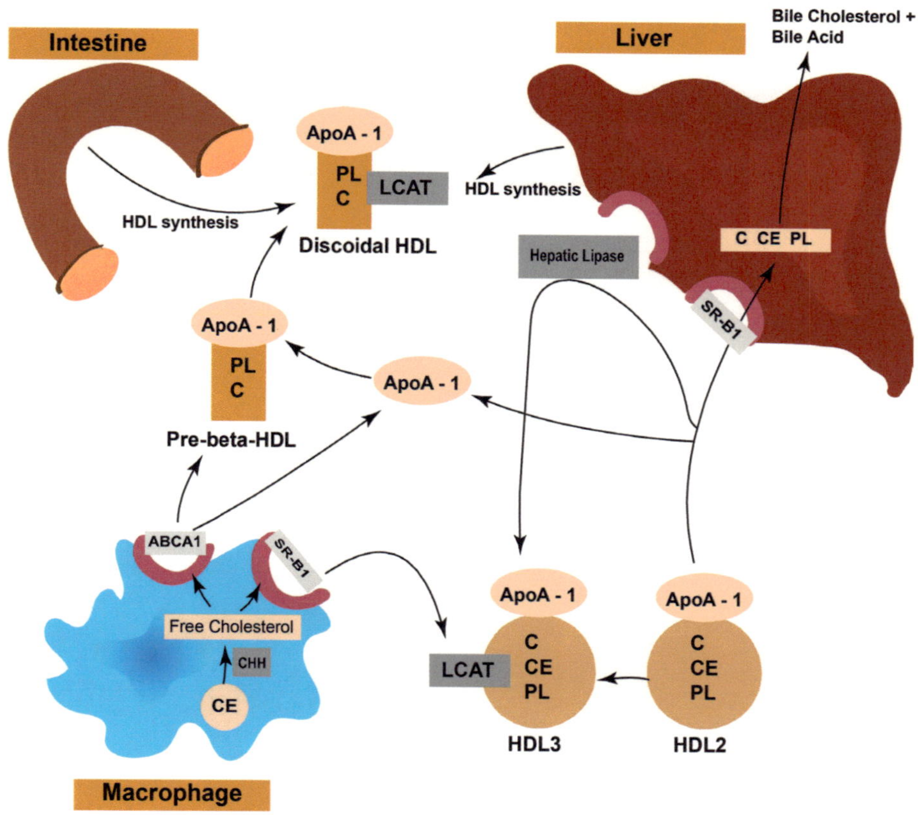

Figure 4.
Reverse cholesterol transport pathway. C, cholesterol; CE, cholesteryl ester; LCAT, lecithin cholesterol ethyl transferase; PL, phospholipid; ApoA-1, apolipoprotein A-1.

Certain disease states interfere with lipid transport pathways, leading to serious disorders. For example, in diabetes mellitus, relative insulin resistance causes under-utilization of VLDLs and chylomicrons, eventually leading to hypertriacylglycerolemia and increased small-density LDLs which promotes atherosclerosis [8]. Among many other roles, insulin inhibits the release of free fatty acids (FFA) from the adipose tissues and suppresses hepatic VLDL secretion into the circulation. These mechanisms come into play in the role of diabetes as a risk factor for CVD including stroke [8].

Furthermore, the inability to suppress VLDL-triglyceride kinetics has been implicated in the pathogenesis of nonalcoholic fatty liver disease [9], a serious complication that leads to CVD, cancer, and liver fibrosis and increases mortality [10].

9. In conclusion

In this short introductory chapter, we provided a brief overview of lipid metabolism highlighting the role of lipids as CVD risk factors, the various types of lipid structure and function as well as the exogenous (intestinal), and the endogenous lipid transport pathways through which fats are transported from the intestines and the liver, respectively, to the peripheral tissues. We also highlighted in some detail the reverse cholesterol transfer pathway via which cholesterol, in the form of cholesterol esters, are transported from the blood vessel walls and other tissues back to the liver for excretion in the bile.

Author details

Angelina Zhyvotovska, Denis Yusupov and Samy I. McFarlane*
State University of New York, Downstate Medical Center, New York, USA

*Address all correspondence to: smcfarlane@downstate.edu

References

[1] Prevention CfDCa. Cholesterol. 2019; https://www.cdc.gov/cholesterol/index/htm [Accessed: October 2, 2019]

[2] Benjamin EJ, Blaha MJ, Chiuve SE, et al. Heart disease and stroke statistics-2017 update: A report from the American Heart Association. Circulation. 2017;**135**(10):e146-e603

[3] Ingelsson E, Massaro JM, Sutherland P, et al. Contemporary trends in dyslipidemia in the Framingham Heart Study. Archives of Internal Medicine. 2009;**169**(3):279-286

[4] Multiple Risk Factor Intervention Trial Research Group. Multiple risk factor intervention trial. Risk factor changes and mortality results. Journal of the American Medical Association. 1982;**248**(12):1465-1477. https://jamanetwork.com/journals/jama/fullarticle/377969

[5] The lipid research clinics coronary primary prevention trial results. I. Reduction in incidence of coronary heart disease. Journal of the American Medical Association. 1984;**251**(3):351-364

[6] Frick MH, Elo O, Haapa K, et al. Helsinki Heart Study: Primary-prevention trial with gemfibrozil in middle-aged men with dyslipidemia. Safety of treatment, changes in risk factors, and incidence of coronary heart disease. The New England Journal of Medicine. 1987;**317**(20):1237-1245

[7] McFarlane SI, Muniyappa R, Francisco R, Sowers JR. Clinical review 145: Pleiotropic effects of statins: Lipid reduction and beyond. The Journal of Clinical Endocrinology and Metabolism. 2002;**87**(4):1451-1458

[8] McFarlane SI, Banerji M, Sowers JR. Insulin resistance and cardiovascular disease. The Journal of Clinical Endocrinology and Metabolism. 2001;**86**(2):713-718

[9] Poulsen MK, Nellemann B, Stodkilde-Jorgensen H, Pedersen SB, Gronbaek H, Nielsen S. Impaired insulin suppression of VLDL-triglyceride kinetics in nonalcoholic fatty liver disease. The Journal of Clinical Endocrinology and Metabolism. 2016;**101**(4):1637-1646

[10] Treeprasertsuk S, Bjornsson E, Enders F, Suwanwalaikorn S, Lindor KD. NAFLD fibrosis score: A prognostic predictor for mortality and liver complications among NAFLD patients. World Journal of Gastroenterology. 2013;**19**(8):1219-1229

Chapter 2

Dyslipidemia and Its Role in the Pathogenesis of Atherosclerotic Cardiovascular Disease: Implications for Evaluation and Targets for Treatment of Dyslipidemia Based on Recent Guidelines

Perry Wengrofsky, Justin Lee and Amgad N. Makaryus

Abstract

The clinical presentations of atherosclerotic disease are the result of a constellation of diverse metabolic and immunologic mechanisms ultimately set into motion by the formation of fatty acid streaks and the accompanying inflammatory cell activation, endothelial damage, smooth muscle proliferation, vascular fibrosis, and end-organ infarction and necrosis. At the heart of atherosclerosis are the byproducts of lipid metabolism, lipoproteins containing triglycerides, phospholipids, and cholesterol, and the changes they undergo that eventually lead to macrophage activation, foam cell formation, and other downstream atherosclerotic changes. Understanding the functionality of cholesterol, triglycerides, and lipoproteins in the cascade of atherosclerotic pathways has tremendous implications on current guidelines for the evaluation and targets in the management of dyslipidemia, and serves as the foundation for future investigations into targets of atherosclerotic therapies.

Keywords: atherosclerosis, dyslipidemia, cardiovascular disease, guidelines

1. Introduction

Atherosclerosis, the pathogenic process of vascular lipid deposition, arterial luminal narrowing, and plaque expansion and instability, represents the major driver of circulatory morbidity and mortality, including myocardial infarction, ischemic cardiomyopathy, transient ischemic attacks, and ischemic and hemorrhagic stroke [1]. The acute and chronic clinical presentations of atherosclerotic disease are the result of a constellation of diverse metabolic and immunologic mechanisms ultimately set into motion by the formation of fatty acid streaks and the accompanying inflammatory cell activation, endothelial damage, smooth muscle proliferation, vascular fibrosis, and end-organ infarction and necrosis [2].

At the heart of atherosclerosis are the byproducts of lipid metabolism, lipoproteins containing triglycerides, phospholipids, and cholesterol, and the changes they undergo that eventually lead to macrophage activation, foam cell formation, and other downstream atherosclerotic changes [3]. Lipoproteins are distinguished by their lipid content, their position in lipid metabolic pathways, and overall atherogenic risk [4, 5]. This chapter will review the role that the various lipoproteins play in the pathophysiology of atherosclerosis as the fundamental triggers and players in the immunologic, inflammatory, and thrombotic processes that characterize the pathogenesis of atherosclerotic cardiovascular disease. Understanding the functionality of cholesterol, triglycerides, and lipoproteins in the cascade of atherosclerotic pathways has tremendous implications on current guidelines for the evaluation and targets in the management of dyslipidemia, and serves as the foundation for future investigations into targets of atherosclerotic therapies.

2. Lipoproteins and apolipoproteins

Lipoproteins are complex plasma particles containing a core of cholesterol esters and triglycerides surrounded by free cholesterol, phospholipids, and apolipoproteins, and are classified based on size, density, and major lipid and apolipoprotein content [6]. Apolipoproteins, structural proteins that bind triglyceride and cholesterol and enable the formation of lipoproteins, enjoy important roles in lipoprotein structure and metabolism by acting as ligands for lipoprotein receptors and activators or inhibitors of enzymes involved in lipoprotein metabolism [6, 7]. The size, structure, and apolipoprotein content of the lipoproteins, namely chylomicrons (CM), very-low-density lipoprotein (VLDL), intermediate-density lipoprotein (IDL), low-density lipoprotein (LDL), high-density lipoprotein (HDL), and lipoprotein(a) [Lp(a)], crystallize into individualized atherosclerotic risk profiles for the specific lipoprotein [8, 9].

2.1 Chylomicrons and chylomicron remnants

CMs, the largest and least dense of the lipoproteins, are triglyceride rich, released from the intestine, and primarily responsible for delivery of dietary cholesterol and triglycerides to peripheral tissue and the liver [6, 10]. Removal of triglycerides from circulating CMs generates CM remnants that possess a considerably higher cholesterol concentration [6, 11]. CMs and CM remnant size is linked to ingested triglyceride levels and the structure is maintained by multiple apolipoproteins, predominantly apolipoprotein B-48 (Apo B-48) [6]. Apo B-48 is synthesized in the intestine, and represents 48% of the amino acids in the peptide sequence of apolipoprotein B-100 (Apo B-100), the apolipoprotein synthesized by the liver and a major apolipoprotein involved in the atherosclerotic pathophysiology [12].

2.2 Very-low-density lipoprotein (VLDL) and intermediate-density lipoprotein (IDL)

Triglyceride consumption by adipose tissue and the resulting cholesterol-rich CM remnants subsequently reach the liver, which reorganizes triglycerides and cholesterol in the form of VLDL that are secreted into circulation and allow for lipoprotein lipase (LPL) mediated absorption of triglycerides by cardiomyocytes, skeletal muscle, and adipose tissue [4, 6]. CMs, CM remnants, and VLDL contain apolipoprotein C (Apo C), specifically Apo C-II, an essential cofactor for LPL, and transposition of triglycerides from circulating lipoproteins to tissue steadily increases the concentration of cholesterol and overall density of the lipoprotein while simultaneously decreasing the size [6, 13]. The apolipoprotein that plays the most atherogenic role of all the apolipoproteins and distinguishes VLDL from chylomicrons and CM remnants is Apo B-100, a major structural apolipoprotein and LDL receptor (LDLR) ligand [6, 14]. VLDL exists as the bridge between the exogenous and endogenous pathways of lipid metabolism, with the lipid content of CM remnants that reach the liver via gastrointestinal absorption at the beginning of the exogenous pathway being repackaged and secreted by hepatocytes as VLDL to initiate the endogenous pathway. IDLs, considered VLDL remnants, are considerably smaller than the antecedent VLDL and exhibit similar apolipoprotein composition, but they have similar triglyceride and cholesterol contents to the CM remnants [4, 14, 15]. The decreased size and cholesterol along with the appropriate apolipoprotein profile of Apo B-100 and Apo-E, another apolipoprotein ligand for the LDLR, make IDL atherogenic, but the primary atherogenic lipoprotein that sets off the cascade of atherosclerotic lipid, immunologic, and inflammatory pathways remains LDL (**Table 1**).

2.3 Low-density lipoprotein (LDL)

LDL, derived from LPL/Apo C-II-mediated triglyceride removal from VLDL and IDL, is the lipoprotein responsible for cholesterol transport to peripheral tissue and the lipoprotein that has been extensively studied and directly implicated in the development of atherosclerosis [4, 5]. With an average size of 18–25 nm, LDL and the predominant apolipoprotein it contains, Apo B-100, undergo oxidation and other molecular modifications that are responsible for endothelial damage, macrophage chemoattraction, and pathologic arterial changes [1, 6, 16]. Individual LDL particles can vary in size, with decreasing or small dense LDL being noticeably more atherogenic than large LDL particles due to susceptibility to oxidation, ease of extravasation and entrapment in the arterial wall, and avidity for binding with vascular wall proteoglycans [6, 16, 17].

The metabolism of LDL, and thus the circulatory availability and arterial wall extravasation ability of LDL, is determined by the quantity of hepatic LDLR, as the concentration of LDL generated from the metabolism of VLDL and IDL is regulated by the amount of IDL that is absorbed into the liver via the LDLR prior to LPL-mediated triglyceride removal [6, 18]. Hepatic levels of LDLR are primarily modulated by hepatocyte cholesterol levels, with adequate cholesterol levels stimulating

Lipoprotein	Size (nm)	Major lipid content	Apolipoproteins
Chylomicron	>75	Triglyceride	Apo B-48, Apo C, ApoE, Apo A-I, A-II, A-IV
Chylomicron remnants	30–75	Triglyceride, cholesterol	Apo B-48, ApoE
VLDL	30–75	Triglyceride	Apo B-100, Apo C, ApoE
IDL	25–35	Triglyceride, cholesterol	Apo B-100, Apo C, ApoE
LDL	<25	Cholesterol	Apo B-100
Lp(a)	30	Cholesterol	Apo B-100, Apo(a)
HDL	<15	Cholesterol, phospholipids	Apo A-1, A-II Apo C, ApoE

Table 1.
Lipoproteins—size, lipid, and apolipoprotein content.

LDLR targeting for degradation by PCSK9, a protein synthesized by hepatocytes that binds the LDLR and promotes lysosomal LDLR degradation [5, 6, 19].

LDL subfraction sizes and the resulting atherogenicity need to be considered when evaluating patients, as therapeutic regimens (such as niacin) have been known to affect LDL particle size. It is also important to realize that while overall cholesterol panel level changes may occur and appear to be in the right direction, it is actually the atherogenicity of the particles specifically of LDL that drives the pathogenesis of atherosclerosis [20]. Analysis, therefore, of LDL subfractions may be an important component of lipid follow-up in patients with complex lipid disorders on combination pharmacologic therapy.

2.4 High-density lipoprotein (HDL)

HDL differs from VLDL, IDL, and LDL in size, lipid, and apolipoprotein content, role in cholesterol metabolic pathways, and antiatherogenic characteristics. HDL is responsible for peripheral cholesterol uptake and delivery to the liver- and cholesterol-derived hormone-producing organs, and it provides important antioxidant and anti-inflammatory functions that can inhibit atherosclerosis [4, 6, 21]. Devoid of Apo B-100 that contributes to LDL oxidation and subsequent macrophage activation, HDL is associated with multiple subtypes of apolipoprotein A (Apo A) that facilitates cholesterol transfer from peripheral tissue and activates lecithin-cholesterol acyltransferance (LCAT), which allows for cholesterol esterification and movement of cholesterol from the HDL surface to the HDL core [6, 22]. After cholesterol uptake from peripheral tissue and macrophages, HDL facilitates transfer to the liver via scavenger receptor class B type I (SR-B1), where the cholesterol can be converted into bile acids for excretion or be directly secreted into bile [21, 23]. The apolipoprotein profile and receptors involved in cholesterol movement from HDL sheds light on some of the physiologic pathways involved in HDL attenuation of atherosclerosis and conversely the highly atherogenic contents and formulation of LDL.

2.5 Lipoprotein A [Lp(a)]

Lp(a) is the lipoprotein formed of a cholesterol-rich LDL molecule and apolipoprotein a [Apo(a)], with levels that are very fluctuant but are generally dependent on the rates of hepatic production of Apo(a) [6, 24]. The Apo-B100 and the Apo(a) are connected via a disulfide bond, and given its size and cholesterol composition essentially identical to that of LDL, Lp(a) is able to extravasate from plasma into the arterial intima and interact with the extracellular matrix through LDL Apo B-100 and Lp(a) [24–26]. In addition to Lp(a), extracellular matrix interactions that facilitate the trapping of cholesterol that sets the table for macrophage uptake and foam cell formation, Lp(a) disrupts fibrinolysis and enhances coagulation, two functions that promote atherosclerotic plaque instability and rupture [24, 27].

3. Lipoproteins and the atherosclerotic thrombo-inflammatory process

3.1 Endothelial changes and regional plaque distribution

Endothelial cells undergo a series of changes, both connected and unrelated to lipoproteins that contribute to the different pathophysiologic mechanisms at play in atherosclerosis and help to explain the typical regional distributions of atherosclerotic lesions.

While LDL and other small and atherogenic lipoproteins undergo oxidative and structural changes that eventually lead to trapping in the arterial intima that recruit macrophages and other inflammatory cells, access to the intima extracellular matrix is spearheaded by endothelial cell dysfunction and damage from oxidative injury in conditions like smoking and hypertension, advanced glycation end products in diabetes mellitus, and regional hemodynamic forces in particular parts of the arterial tree [1, 28]. Oxidative insults to the endothelium impair production of nitric oxide (NO), the potent modulator of vascular tone and inhibitor of the proliferation of vascular smooth muscle cells (VSMCs), and exhibits important roles in the prevention of LDL oxidation and leukocyte extravasation from the bloodstream to arterial intima [29]. Additional chemical mediators of endothelial dysfunction include endothelin-1 (ET1) that interacts with NO in the regulation of arterial tone, signals changes in endothelial expression of adhesion molecules, and recruits important inflammatory cells such as macrophages while simultaneously regulating extracellular matrix enzymes that contribute to intimal alterations [1, 30].

The endothelial changes that best illuminate the regional pathophysiology of atherosclerosis are not the different levels of NO and other molecular signals, but the regional reorganization of endothelial phenotypes in reaction to local hemodynamic forces. Atherosclerotic plaques generally form at areas of arterial curvature and bifurcation, the locations in the arterial circulation where there are typical patterns of elevated shear stress [31]. Endothelial cells in regions of higher shear stress display a cuboidal morphology, higher cell turnover, and impaired endothelial barrier function that collectively promotes lipoprotein and inflammatory cell migration, in comparison to endothelial cells in arterial beds with more favorable hemodynamics that exhibit ellipsoidal morphology, coaxial alignment, and an endothelial glycocalyx that protects against lipoprotein extravasation [31–33].

While the size, oxidative profiles, and atherogenic risk of the lipoproteins, most significantly LDL and Apo B-100, are the primary drivers of atherosclerosis, critical endothelial changes that further exacerbate the migration of lipoproteins, leukocytes, VSMCs, and fibroblasts are fundamental to the generation of plaques and the clinical consequences of plaque expansion and rupture.

3.2 Initiation of the atherosclerotic plaque: foam cell formation

With continued endothelial compromise in regions of arterial curvature and bifurcation, circulating LDL, and to a lesser degree VLDL and IDL, increasingly migrate from the plasma and are retained in the extracellular matrix of the tunica intima [34, 35]. Subendothelial accumulation of LDL and VLDL remnants precipitates endothelial activation of the nuclear factor kappa B (NF-κB) pathway that enhances endothelial expression of adhesion proteins such as VCAM-1 and P-selection and pro-inflammatory receptors and cytokines that promote monocyte migration [32, 34, 36, 37]. As LDL, VLDL, VLDL remnants, IDL, and Lp(a) collect in the arterial intima, Apo B-100, most significantly in LDL, undergoes oxidation to ox-LDL, a potent ligand of macrophage scavenger receptors [1, 5, 24, 38]. Endothelial activation and upregulation of adhesion molecules enables monocyte rolling, activation, and transendothelial migration where they differentiate from monocytes into macrophages [34, 39]. Retained ox-LDL interacts with two macrophage receptors, class A and B scavenger receptors, and in distinct contrast to cholesterol absorbed via the LDLR by the macrophage, ox-LDL does not cause a negative feedback on scavenger receptor expression, perpetuating continued ox-LDL and cholesterol uptake, resulting in the entrapment of newly formed foam cells in the arterial intima secondary to compromised mobility [1, 34, 39, 40].

Despite the predominance of LDL in the cycle of endothelial damage, macrophage absorption, foam cell formation, and inflammatory transduction, VLDL and Lp(a) play important roles in endothelial activation [4, 24]. Endothelial cell exposure to the triglycerides of VLDL stimulates expression of selectins and other proteins that promote monocyte entry into the arterial intima, and oxidized VLDL increases expression of plasminogen activator inhibitor 1 (PAI-1), a protein that attenuates plasminogen conversion to plasmin and thus plasmin-mediated dismantling of cholesterol aggregates [4, 41, 42]. Lp(a) interactions with certain macrophage surface integrin proteins promote monocyte extravasation and upon macrophage absorption, upregulates expression of IL-1, tumor necrosis factor (TNF) and monocyte chemoattractant protein (MCP-1) that recruits additional macrophages, resulting in formation of more foam cells [24, 43].

3.3 Plaque development: inflammatory cells and smooth muscle cells

In addition to uptake by macrophages, ox-LDL acts as an omnipotent chemokine that induces the activity of multiple immunologic pathways and leads to the migration and activation of additional monocytes and other inflammatory cells and VSMCs [1, 32, 44]. While LDL, VLDL remnants, IDL, and Lp(a) retention leads to foam cell formation as the integral first step in plaque development, subsequent leukocyte adhesion and extravasation promotes clearance of foam cells and apoptotic cell debris from dendritic cells and T cells via a complicated interaction between the innate and adaptive immune systems [33, 45–47]. Atherosclerotic lesion macrophages differentiating into inflammatory M1 macrophages present antigens to T cells, with resulting T cell activation and release of pro-inflammatory cytokines such as IL-1 and IL-6, inducing local lesion inflammation, further foam cell formation, and subsequent foam cell apoptosis and necrosis (**Figure 1**) [1, 48, 49].

In a similar pattern to macrophages, foam cells undergo phagocytosis by dendritic cells, where antigen presentation to T cells promotes release of pro-inflammatory cytokine, and continued phagocytosis compromises dendritic cell mobility resulting in dendritic foam cell formation [45, 50, 51].

The cascade of endothelial dysfunction, lipoprotein accumulation, and inflammatory pathways results in dramatic changes in VSMC physiology [32, 52]. Native arterial media VSMCs are activated and undergo proliferation, migration, and phenotypic switching that ultimately plays the most critical roles in atherosclerotic plaque stability or vulnerability [52–54]. VSMC proliferation and migration results in increased production of extracellular matrix components, such as proteoglycans and elastin, that attempts to compensate for the inward architectural distortions caused by subendothelial lipoprotein accumulation, causing outward vascular remodeling [32, 34, 55]. Collagen production by VSMCs is the most critical component in the development of the fibrous cap in atherosclerotic plaques, with TGF-β released from plaque macrophages signaling VSMC proliferation [34, 56, 57].

3.4 HDL and plaque development

The multifaceted pathways of atherosclerotic plaque development and the role LDL and other Apo B-100 lipoproteins serve as a template for the important roles and diverse protective mechanisms and functions of HDL in the pathogenesis of atherosclerosis. Oxidation of Apo-B100 and the resulting accumulation and macrophage phagocytosis of LDL and other lipoproteins can be mitigated by the antioxidant activity of HDL, with its major apolipoproteins, Apo A-I and Apo A-II, and HDL-associated enzymes such as paraoxonase possessing antioxidant activity [21, 58, 59]. Resolving oxidative stress allows HDL to normalize endothelial function

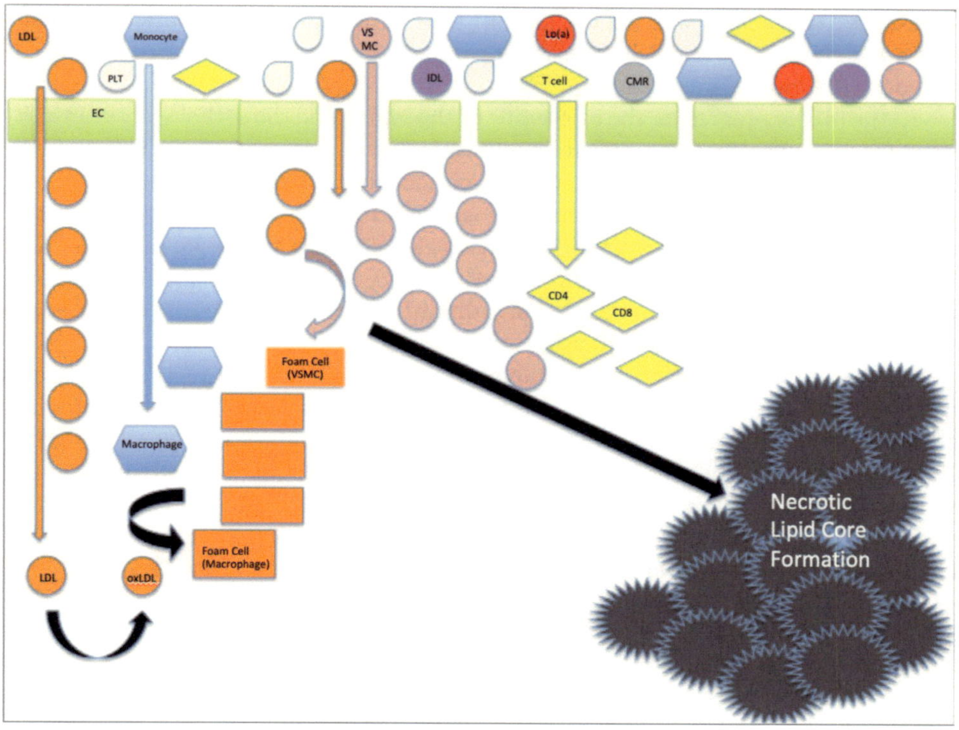

Figure 1.
Small lipoproteins, most prominent LDL, penetrate the dysfunctional endothelial barrier and accumulate in the arterial intima. LDL (Apo B-100 apolipoprotein component) undergoes oxidation to ox-LDL, which triggers inflammatory cascade promoting migration of monocytes, VSMCs, and CD4 and CD8 T cells. ox-LDL undergoes phagocytosis by macrophages (and VSMCs) to generate foam cells. Insufficient clearance of apoptotic foam and inflammatory cells causes steady accumulation of subendothelial lipid necrotic core, which serves as central component of developing atherosclerotic plaque.

by restoring production of NO [23, 60, 61]. HDL disrupts monocyte migration into the arterial intima via inhibition of endothelial cell adhesion protein expression, the fundamental first step in the formation of foam cells [62, 63]. HDL also inhibits VSMC migration and mitigates coagulation system and platelet activation, which come more into play in acute plaque rupture [4, 21, 64].

The major roles of HDL in atherosclerotic plaque development are inhibiting foam cell formation by promoting cholesterol transfer from macrophages and attenuating local lesion inflammation. In a pattern similar to normal reverse cholesterol transport from peripheral tissue to hepatocytes, HDL can remove cholesterol from macrophages and foam cells in the arterial intima via passive aqueous diffusion or cholesterol transporters, such as ATP-binding cassette transporters A1 (ABCA1) and G1 (ABCG1) and scavenger-receptor BI (SR-BI) that utilize the cholesterol concentration gradient [34, 65, 66]. HDL inhibits the M1 phenotype inflammatory macrophages that dominate in atherosclerotic plaques and present antigens to T cells while promoting M2 anti-inflammatory macrophages and modulating apoptosis of foam cells via antiapoptotic signaling pathways [67–69].

4. Atherosclerotic plaque progression, stability, and acute rupture

4.1 Plaque progression: fibrous cap and necrotic lipid core

Smooth muscle proliferation within the atherosclerotic plaque is characterized by the production of a subendothelial complex extracellular matrix making up the fibrous cap that acts to wall off the inflammatory and highly thrombotic lesion collection of cholesterol and cell debris that results from immune-mediated apoptosis and destruction of foam cells [1, 70, 71].

As the plaque progresses, the thickening of the intima and the pathologic expansion into the lumen displays areas of distinct cellular and lipid content, with the mature fibroatheroma consisting of an acellular lipid necrotic core of cell debris [71, 76]. The lipid component of the necrotic core consists of foam cells and newly free cholesterol from apoptotic macrophages that have been ineffectively cleared by efferocytosis [1, 71–73]. The necrotic lipid core can undergo steady expansion with resulting plaque enlargement and decreasing arterial lumen caliber due to diminished clearance capacity of cholesterol by VSMCs and advanced plaque macrophages [34, 74].

The steady accumulation of free cholesterol and lipid material alongside necrotic cellular products from apoptosis generates a continuous release of pro-inflammatory stimuli that further promote additional foam cell destruction, a vicious cycle that is contained by the thick collagenous fibrous cap [71, 75]. Vascular remodeling counterbalances this continuous inflammatory process defined by intimal accumulation and lesion expansion, which minimizes protrusion into the lumen and mitigates clinical symptomology over the lifetime of the lesion (**Figure 2**) [34, 71, 76].

4.2 Stable and vulnerable plaques

The structural makeup of the plaque and relationship between fibrous cap thickness, lipid and necrotic core size, inflammatory activity, and overlying endothelial integrity translate to overall atherosclerotic plaque stability and risk of plaque compromise.

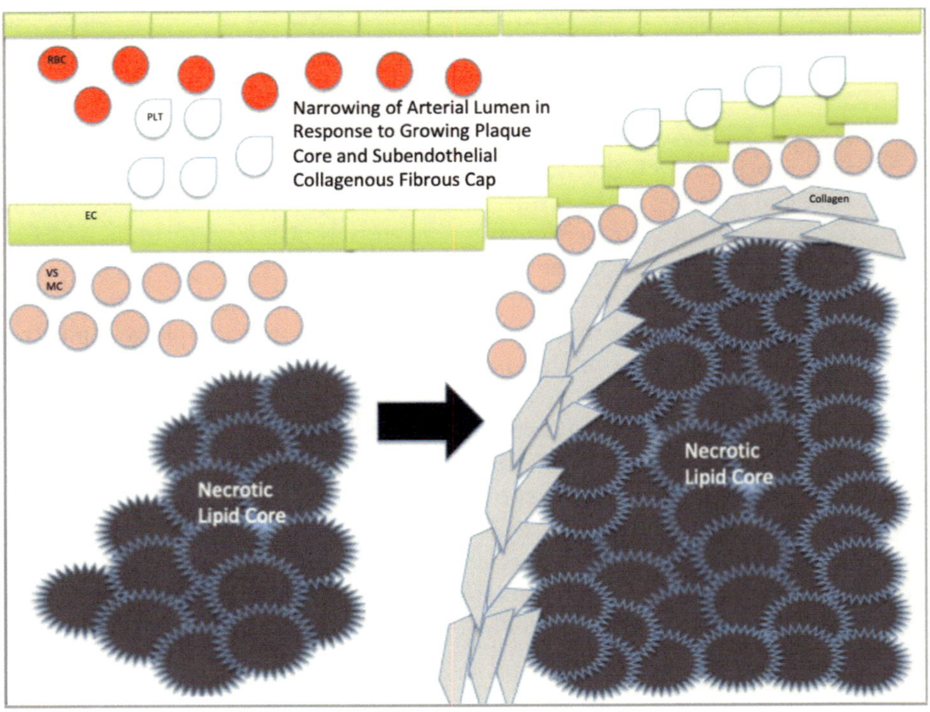

Figure 2.
Steady development of the necrotic lipid core leads to subendothelial expansion, which over time narrows the diameter of the arterial lumen. VSMC migration, proliferation, and activation lead to deposition of fibrous collagenous extracellular matrix material to create the fibrous cap of the atherosclerotic plaque. Overlying dysfunction endothelial changes and breaks in the barrier allow for exposure of the contents of the cap and core to interact with serum cells and proteins, leading to platelet adherence to intact but vulnerable plaques.

In stable atherosclerotic plaques, low-grade inflammation enables VSMC enrichment, which increases the percentage of the plaque that is made up of the collagenous fibrous cap [77, 78]. In general, the lines of demarcation between more stable and more vulnerable plaques tend to center around the ratio between the solid fibrous tissue and the extracellular lipid necrotic tissue, with stable and clinically silent plaques typically displaying thick fibrous caps and minimal to no extracellular lipid and necrotic foam cell debris [77, 79, 80]. While fibrous cap thickness and strength is a critical determinant of overall plaque stability, the fibrous tissue laid down by VSMC in the subendothelial part of the arterial intima is in a constant state of balance between collagen synthesis and degradation mediated by inflammatory cytokines that upregulate the expression of matrix metalloproteinases (MMPs) [1, 78, 81, 82]. MMPs can degrade fibrillar collagen, proteoglycans, and elastin over time, and the resulting thinning and structural compromise of the fibrous cap transitions the stable plaque to a vulnerable and high-risk plaque [77, 78, 83].

In parallel to the changes in the fibrous cap are dynamic swings in inflammatory conditions in the necrotic lipid core, where increasing levels of VSMC and macrophage apoptosis not only decrease the net number of cells that can synthesize collagen and other stabilizing extracellular matrix components but also release additional inflammatory cytokines that can further destabilize the plaque [78, 84]. Similar to the roles played in plaque development, T cells, both T helper CD4 T cells and T cytotoxic CD8 cells, contribute to plaque destabilization via a perpetual loop of macrophage and T cell recruitment, lipid uptake, foam cell formation, antigen presentation, apoptosis, and lipid necrotic core expansion [78, 85, 86].

4.3 Rupture and erosion of vulnerable plaques and acute thrombosis

The nonresolving inflammatory processes of lipoprotein accumulation, foam cell formation, and immunologic activation leads to fibrocellular organization of the plaque, with the plaque becoming increasingly unstable and prone to rupture and acute thrombosis via fibrous cap thinning and lipid necrotic core expansion [34, 77, 87]. The fibrous cap is thinned and weakened by MMPs, and disruption of the collagenous cap and the overlying endothelium leads to exposure of the highly thrombogenic and coagulable lipid necrotic core [1, 88]. Atherosclerotic plaques, prior to any sort of structural compromise, are congregated by platelets that attach to the dysfunctional endothelium of the plaque, and can participate in plaque-associated thrombosis with and without rupture or erosion [88, 89].

Ruptured and eroded plaques trigger a rapid and dramatic thrombotic and coagulation process, with activated platelets adhering to the exposed subendothelial collagen of the thin fibrous cap via interactions between von Willebrand factor (vWF) and glycoprotein (GP) Ib-V-IX, with adherent-activated platelets aggregating via GP IIb/IIIa complexes [90–92]. After adhesion, activated-aggregated platelets release granules containing thromboxane A2, adenosine diphosphate (ADP), and other pro-thrombotic and pro-inflammatory cytokines that recruit inflammatory cells and amplify the platelet response (**Figure 3**) [1, 90, 93].

Alongside platelet activation and thrombus formation is activation of the coagulation system, with tissue factor (TF) receptors in the plaque binding circulating factor VII(a) and triggering the extrinsic coagulation pathway to produce thrombin [90, 94, 95]. Thrombin, a strong platelet agonist via protease-activated receptor (PARs)-1 and 4, converts fibrinogen to fibrin for clot stabilization while simultaneously driving its own positive feedback loops through activation of factor XI and other factors in the intrinsic coagulation pathway [90, 96, 97].

The constellation of plaque rupture, platelet activation and aggregation, and coagulation system stimulation results in the formation of a thrombus on an

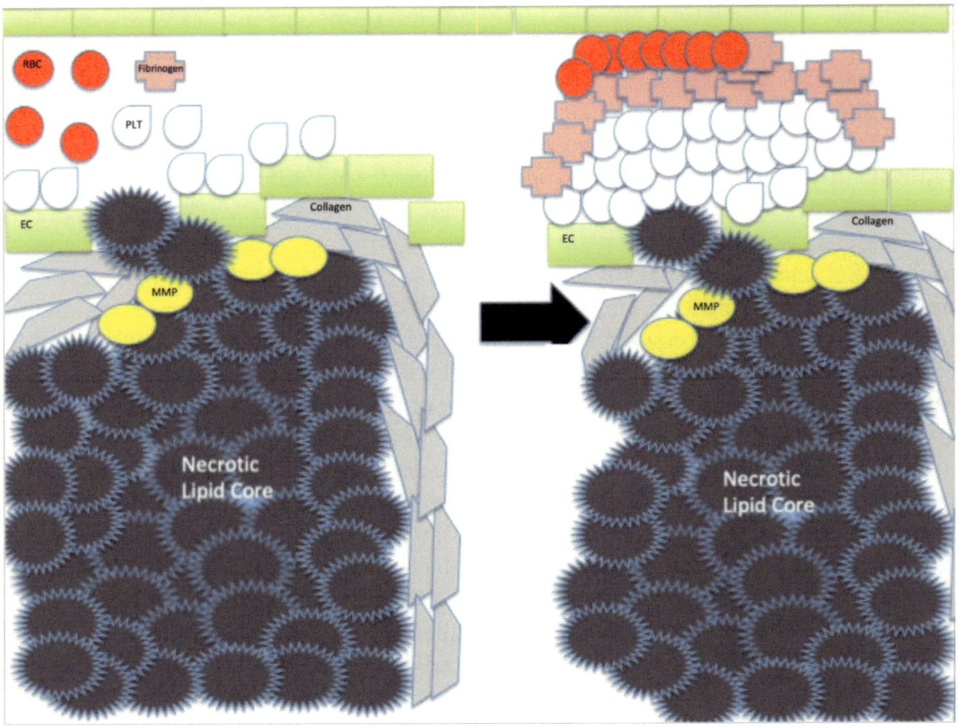

Figure 3.
Rupture or erosion of the plaque's fibrous cap enables exposure of highly thrombogenic and coagulable necrotic lipid core content to circulating platelets and coagulation factors. Acute atherothrombosis results with dramatic aggregation and activation of platelets and coagulation factors, resulting in acute occlusion of the implicated arterial tree and downstream tissue ischemia and necrosis.

atherosclerotic plaque, causing partial to complete obstruction of the arterial lumen, which has already been narrowed steadily over time by plaque progression [1, 34, 90]. Postmortem pathological examination of these atherosclerotic plaque thrombi show a directional morphology that highlights the stepwise process of thrombus formation, with white platelet-rich heads adjacent to the focus of plaque rupture, with red extensions from the white platelet head to the distal arterial wall encompassing the fibrin and red blood cells that accumulate secondary to diminished blood flow from the obstructive thrombus [90, 98, 99].

5. Atherosclerotic cardiovascular disease: presentation, evaluation, and management

5.1 Atherosclerotic cardiovascular disease (ASCVD)

ASCVD is the clinical manifestation of atherosclerosis and atherothrombosis, the resulting symptomology and physical findings of acute and chronic end-organ ischemia and infarction from the pathophysiologic thrombo-inflammatory process of atherogenesis initiated by cholesterol and lipoprotein accumulation in the arterial intima. Public health appreciation and scientific evidence for the role of dyslipidemia in the progression of ASCVD has served as the impetus for organizations throughout the United States, Canada, and Europe to develop guidelines for evaluation and management of dyslipidemia and ASCVD [100–102]. Furthermore, the severity and associated morbidity and mortality of the clinical manifestations of ASCVD, including ischemic heart disease, such as stable angina, unstable angina, non-ST-elevation myocardial infarction (NSTEMI), and ST-elevation myocardial infarction (STEMI), peripheral artery disease (PAD), and cerebrovascular disease, both intracranial and extracranial, have prompted the development of condition specific guidelines for primary prevention, acute management, and secondary prevention [103–114]. Guidelines for management of dyslipidemia in the context of ASCVD are centered on the presence of pre-existing ASCVD, age, and underlying comorbidities, most prominently diabetes.

5.2 Coronary artery disease/ischemic heart disease

In the context of ASCVD, coronary artery disease (CAD), also referred to as ischemic heart disease (IHD), covers a spectrum of acute and chronic conditions resulting from myocardial oxygen demand and supply mismatch, generally caused by atherosclerotic disease of native coronary arteries, both fixed lesions and acute atherothrombosis [107, 115, 116].

Stable angina pectoris is a syndrome of recurrent and intermittent episodes of chest pain during instances of increased myocardial oxygen demand and insufficient oxygen supply from flow-limiting atherosclerotic coronary lesions [116, 117]. Stable angina is the initial clinical manifestation of nearly half of all patients with CAD, and given the high rates of myocardial infarction in patients with stable angina, extensive guidelines on workup and management, including stress testing, coronary calcium scoring by computed tomography, and cardiac catheterization and revascularization, to mitigate the risk of future major cardiovascular events [107, 117, 118].

Acute coronary syndrome (ACS), the acute manifestations of CAD, include unstable angina (UA), non-ST-elevation myocardial infarction (NSTEMI), and ST-elevation myocardial infarction (STEMI) are distinguished primarily by the absence of presence of electrocardiographic (EKG) changes and troponin elevation [115, 119]. The pathophysiology that differentiates stable angina from ACS is acute plaque rupture or erosion that results in the acute worsening of coronary artery flow, with subsequent symptomatic, electrocardiographic, and biochemical clinical findings ranging from moderate to severe chest pain all the way to acute cardiogenic shock and cardiac arrest [120, 121]. Myocardial infarction (MI), both NSTEMI and STEMI, caused by acute atherothrombotic disease of an eroded or ruptured plaque, is classified as a type I MI [115, 122]. It is distinguished from other etiologies of cardiomyocyte damage, troponin elevation, and EKG changes such as other acute stressors such as anemia, sepsis, or tachyarrhythmia that cause oxygen demand-supply mismatch (type 2 MI), sudden cardiac death with symptoms suggestive of MI but no blood specimen available for troponin analysis (type 3 MI), type 4 MI as a complication of percutaneous coronary intervention (PCI), and type 5 MI as a complication of coronary artery bypass grafting (CABG) [115, 122–124]. The severity of clinical presentation, along with the acute and long-term risk after adequate management of ACS, has led to countless clinical trials and guideline recommendations on the acute management, involving antiplatelet and anticoagulation therapy, thrombolysis, PCI, and CABG [104–106, 125–127].

5.3 Cerebrovascular disease

Intracranial and extracranial atherosclerotic disease, the drivers of ischemic cerebrovascular accident (CVA/stroke), can be the initial manifestation of atherosclerotic cardiovascular disease or can present concurrently with atherosclerotic disease in other arterial beds, including CAD or PAD [111, 112, 128]. Stroke is classified as either hemorrhagic or ischemic, with hemorrhagic stroke accounting for less than 20% of all strokes, with pathophysiology centered upon ruptured cerebral vessels that have been damaged secondary to longstanding hypertension and amyloid angiopathy [129, 130]. While acute ischemic stroke can be caused by thromboembolic disease, particularly in the setting of atrial fibrillation, acute ischemic stroke is generally caused by acute thrombosis at the site of a cerebral atherosclerotic lesion, with neurologic motor and sensory manifestations in the anatomical distributions innervated by the affected region of the brain [112, 128, 131, 132]. In similar patterns to coronary artery disease, atherosclerotic cerebrovascular disease carries severely high rates of morbidity and mortality, with extensive evidence from clinical trials and guidelines directing highly time sensitive interventions, including thrombolysis and thrombectomy, and the general recommendations for primary and secondary prevention, including stroke-related treatment of dyslipidemia [112, 113, 131, 133, 134].

5.4 Peripheral artery disease

While clinicians classically associated peripheral artery disease (PAD) with lower extremity atherosclerotic disease, PAD, also referred to as peripheral vascular disease (PVD), encompasses atherosclerotic symptoms and disease of all non-coronary and non-cerebrovascular arterial trees, including the upper and lower extremities, renal, mesenteric, and aneurysms of the abdominal aorta and its branching vessels [103, 108, 135]. The pathophysiology and the clinical presentation of PAD are directly related to the organ system or extremity perfused by the affected arterial tree, and similar to the contrast in stable angina versus acute coronary syndrome, the symptomology can be both acute and chronic.

Lower extremity PAD can manifest in different ways, with the classical symptom of claudication affecting a very small to large portion of the lower extremity, with the affected area directly related to chronic arterial lumen narrowing from local atherosclerotic lesions and the proximal or distal positioning of the plaque [103, 136]. The most acute presentation of PAD is acute limb ischemia, the sudden loss of limb perfusion with associated symptoms typically of severe pain, can be caused by thromboembolism but more commonly is secondary to acute atherothrombosis from a ruptured or eroded atherosclerotic plaque [137–139]. Acute limb ischemia is distinct from critical limb ischemia (CLI), with CLI being classified alongside chronic PAD as CLI progresses over several weeks to months, with clinical symptoms of ischemic extremity pain at rest and/or development of ischemic tissue loss such as non-healing ulcers or gangrene [140–142]. The diagnosis and management, both in the acute and chronic setting, involves assessing pulse and blood pressure differences between upper and lower extremities using the ankle-brachial index, vascular imaging, and revascularization, including thrombolysis, endovascular repair, or open surgical correction [103, 108, 143–145].

Non-lower extremity PAD, including renal artery disease, mesenteric arterial disease, and aortic and branching vessel aneurysms represent additional manifestations of atherosclerotic cardiovascular disease with similar presentations of the acute and chronic natures.

Atherosclerotic renal arterial disease classically manifests as chronic renal disease, primarily presenting as a common cause of secondary hypertension from increased activation of the renin-angiotensin-aldosterone system [108, 146, 147]. Additionally, atherosclerotic renal arterial disease can appear as ischemic nephropathy with renal parenchymal disease and manifestations of renal failure from chronic hypoperfusion, microvascular damage, and tubulointerstitial injury [146, 148]. Atherosclerotic renal arterial disease should be considered in patients with accelerated, resistant, or malignant hypertension with new onset acute renal failure or congestive heart failure, evaluated with renovascular imaging such as duplex ultrasonography and angiography, and appropriately managed with either medical therapy or revascularization, both endovascular and surgical [108, 149–151]. Mesenteric ischemia can likewise present with chronic and acute symptoms, with chronic symptoms of abdominal pain with eating, classically referred to as intestinal or postprandial angina and representative of oxygen supply demand mismatch secondary to increased intestinal metabolic activity and diminished mesenteric arterial perfusion from underlying atherosclerosis flow-limiting lesions [108, 152]. Acute obstructive intestinal ischemia can be secondary to thromboembolism or to acute thrombosis of a ruptured or eroded atherosclerotic plaque, presenting classically with severe abdominal pain out of proportion to the physical exam, a critical condition that can result in bowel necrosis and acute abdomen [153, 154]. Given the associated morbidity and mortality, particularly of acute mesenteric ischemia, rapid general and vascular surgery consultation, with prompt diagnostic imaging and intervention is critical for appropriate evaluation and management [108, 155, 156].

Important components of the pathophysiology that promotes arterial lumen narrowing in atherosclerosis, namely chronic inflammation and extracellular matrix degradation initiated by oxidized lipoprotein accumulation, are critical processes that contribute to development of abdominal aortic aneurysms (AAA) [157]. While the precise mechanism of atherosclerosis and its relationship to the development of aneurysms of the abdominal aorta and its branch vessels is yet unclear, the high overlap of risk factors and similar pathophysiologic processes between the two conditions has prompted development of guidelines for monitoring and management of dyslipidemia in patients with known AAA, along with appropriate surveillance imaging for assessment of aneurysmal diameter [108, 158].

6. Evaluation, management, and prevention of dyslipidemia and atherosclerosis

6.1 Cholesterol monitoring, LDL, and evolution of dyslipidemia cardiovascular risk algorithms

While the Apo B-100 cholesterol carrying lipoproteins all play roles in the pathogenesis of atherosclerosis through the critical initiating steps of arterial intima lipid accumulation and foam cell formation, cholesterol monitoring and assessment of atherosclerotic cardiovascular risk has centered around surveillance and management of serum LDL and LDL-cholesterol (LDL-C) levels based on the abundant evidence available from epidemiologic and genetic hypercholesterolemia studies, and randomized controlled trials [5, 159]. IDL, Lp(a), small VLDL, and VLDL remnants all possess the requisite diameter (<70 nm) and apolipoprotein profile (Apo B-100) to freely enter the arterial intima, undergo oxidation, and trigger macrophage phagocytosis, but LDL and LDL-C have been demonstrated to be the most atherogenic of the lipoproteins, with probability of LDL retention and risk of progressive plaque development increasing in parallel with LDL and LDL-C levels in dose-dependent manners [5, 35, 159]. Genetic studies of patients with familial hypercholesterolemia (FH), a spectrum of autosomal co-dominant disorders with different loss or gain of function mutations involving genes involved in LDL metabolism, most commonly presenting as a loss of function mutation of the LDLR, carries a markedly increased risk for ASCVD in heterozygous FH patients, with the rare patients who are homozygous FH developing ASCVD as early as childhood and adolescence [5, 160, 161]. Large epidemiologic studies and meta-analyses have also demonstrated linear associations between LDL-C levels and risk of CAD death [5, 162]. The most compelling evidence for the association between LDL-C and ASCVD comes from the library of evidence from randomized controlled clinical trials showing risk reduction of major cardiovascular events and progression of atherosclerotic plaques proportional to the decrease in LDL-C levels from statin and non-statin therapies [5, 163, 164]. Additionally, LDL subfraction sizes and the resulting atherogenicity need to be considered when evaluated patients, as studies have shown that while overall cholesterol panel levels may be ameliorated with therapy, it is the atherogenicity of the particles, specifically of LDL, that drives the pathogenesis of atherosclerosis [20]. Analysis, therefore, of LDL subfractions is likely an important component of lipid panel monitoring in these patients.

In parallel to the clinical studies and trials demonstrating the relationship between LDL, LDL-C, and ASCVD were the development of algorithms for the appropriate assessment and stratification of cardiovascular risk based on serum lipid profiles and other modifiable and non-modifiable cardiovascular risk factors, including age, gender, family history, smoking, obesity, and hypertension [165, 166]. Multiple ASCVD risk algorithms exist both in the US and Europe, and include the Framingham Risk Score (FRS), the Reynolds Risk Score (RRS), the Systematic Coronary Risk Evaluation (SCORE), the QRisk2, and the American College of Cardiology/American Heart Association arteriosclerotic cardiovascular disease risk estimator (AC/AHA-ASCVD) which has become the benchmark for risk stratification and clinical decision-making on cholesterol therapies [167].

Prior to the assessment of ASCVD risk and decisions on dyslipidemia therapy guidelines and recommendations for screening of cholesterol levels in adult patients who are asymptomatic and without history of ASCVD are employed. Differences exist in screening recommendations in the American, Canadian, and European dyslipidemia guidelines that were published in 2018, 2016, and 2016, respectively [100–102]. Canadian and European guidelines propose that dyslipidemia screening be considered for men at or older than 40 years of age, but diverge on the initial age for women, with Canadian guidelines recommending at or older than 40 years of age, and European guidelines recommending at or older than 50 years of age [100, 102]. According to American guidelines, as recommended in the recently published "2018 AHA/ACC/ACCVPR/AAPA/ABC/ACPM/ADA/AGS/APhA/ASPC/NLA/PCNA Guideline on the Management of Blood Cholesterol," screening for LDL-C and non LDL-C can begin in adults as early as 20 years of age, or childhood or adolescence for patients with a history of FH [101].

6.2 Dyslipidemia: primary prevention of ASCVD

Compared to prior US cholesterol guidelines, the new 2018 ACC/AHA [101] guideline allows for more personalized targeted care for patients. By providing a guided approach to treatment for clinicians, they and their patients are given the tools necessary to understand and manage their risk related to cholesterol. Additionally, these revised guidelines highlight the importance of the "clinician-patient discussion." This patient risk discussion should include a review of risk enhancers to arrive at an appropriate share decision-making approach that addresses the patient's values in terms of cost, potential for benefit, adverse effects, and drug-drug interactions.

The 2018 ACC/AHA guideline recommends that primary management of dyslipidemia for the primary prevention of ASCVD be considered for adult patients based on LDL-C levels and specific high-risk patient characteristics, most prominently a comorbid diagnosis of DM.

Anticholesterol therapy is indicated for adult patients with LDL-C greater than 190 mg/dL or for selected patients with moderately high LDL-C levels greater than

160 mg/dL and a family history of premature ASCVD such as MI or CVA before 55 years of age in a first-degree male relative or before 65 years of age in a first-degree female relative (**Figure 4**).

Patients without LDL-C > 190 mg/dL or without LDL-C > 160 mg/dL and significant family history of premature ASCVD are categorized based on the presence of DM and their 10-year ASCVD risk as estimated by their ASCVD score.

Special attention is paid to DM in the context of the primary prevention of ASCVD as DM is a major risk factor for ASCVD and contributes to and accelerates the pathogenesis of atherosclerosis through multiple and diverse mechanisms [168, 169]. DM amplifies the immune response of key inflammatory cells, most critically macrophages, into the arterial intima in response to lipoprotein accumulation, and promotes the instability of atherosclerotic plaques by increasing the size of the necrotic lipid cores [169–171]. For adult patients, age 40–75 years, with DM, current guidelines recommend initiation of moderate-intensity statin therapy with consideration for possible high-intensity statin therapy depending on patient's individualized risk assessment.

For adult patients, age 40–75 years, without DM, decisions on lifestyle modifications and statin therapy are guided by the 10-year ASCVD risk as estimated by

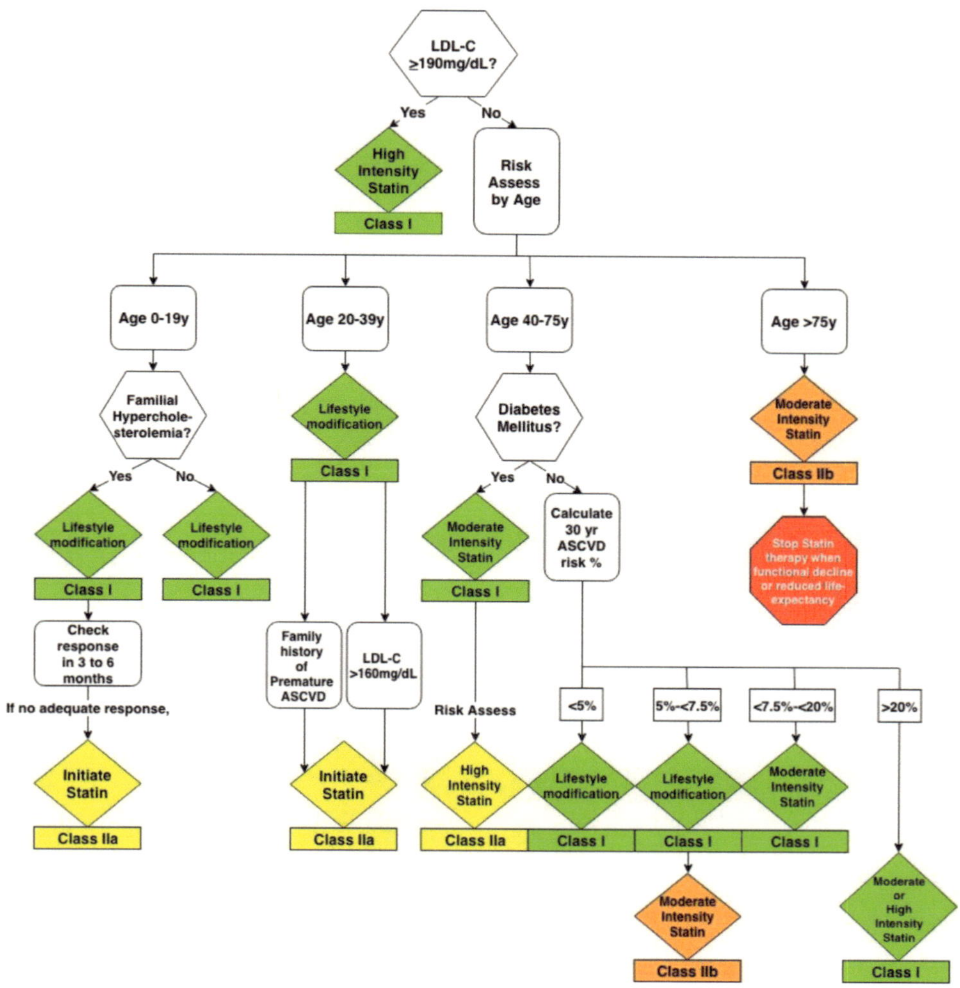

Figure 4.
Management algorithm of dyslipidemia for primary prevention of ASCVD (adapted from 2018 AHA/ACC/ACCVPR/AAPA/ABC/ACPM/ADA/AGS/APhA/ASPC/NLA/PCNA Guideline on the Management of Blood Cholesterol).

the patient's ASCVD score, with patients with a 10-year ASCVD risk score >7.5% qualifying for moderate-intensity statin therapy, and for patient' with a 10-year ASCVD risk score >20% qualifying for moderate to high-intensity statin therapy. Beyond the 10-year ASCVD risk score, clinician-patient discussions of dyslipidemia and primary risk prevention should consider multiple factors, including patient preference, likelihood of statin side effects, prospective benefit of intensive lifestyle modifications, and presence or absence of risk-enhancing factors. Important risk-enhancing factors to consider include metabolic syndrome, chronic kidney disease, chronic inflammatory or infectious conditions such as rheumatologic disease or HIV/AIDs, high-risk race or ethnicity, family history of premature ASCVD, and presence of lipid levels or biomarkers associated with increased ASCVD risk such as elevated Lp(a).

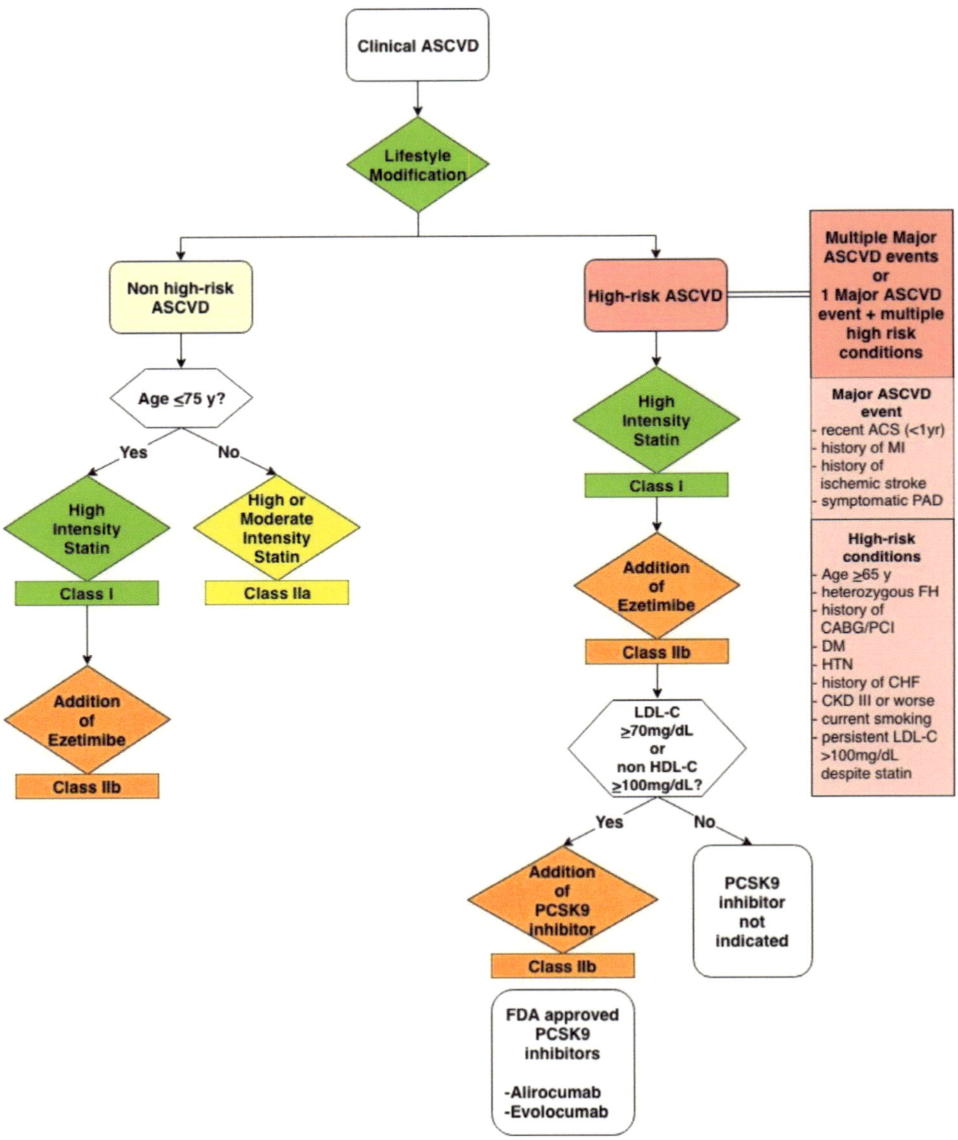

Figure 5.
Management algorithm of dyslipidemia for secondary prevention of ASCVD (adapted from 2018 AHA/ACC/ACCVPR/AAPA/ABC/ACPM/ADA/AGS/APhA/ASPC/NLA/PCNA Guideline on the Management of Blood Cholesterol).

6.3 Dyslipidemia: secondary prevention of ASCVD

Management of dyslipidemia for the secondary prevention of ASCVD is centered on encouragement of intensive healthy lifestyle modifications and risk assessment for future ASCVD. Patients with high or very high-risk ASCVD are those with multiple major ASCVD events or one major ASCVD event and multiple high-risk conditions. Major ASCVD events include ACS within last 12 months, MI, ischemia CVA, PAD with claudication and ABI < 0.85, and PAD with previous revascularization or amputation. High-risk conditions are similar to the risk-enhancing factors that were considered for the management of dyslipidemia in the context of primary prevention of ASCVD, and include age > 65, history of CABG or PCI outside of the major ASCVD events, DM, hypertension, chronic kidney disease, current smoking status, congestive heart failure, and persistently elevated LDL-C above 100 mg/dL despite maximal tolerate dose of statin therapy and ezetimibe, an anticholesterol drug that decreased small intestine absorption of cholesterol (**Figure 5**).

For patients with the aforementioned high-risk conditions who are on the maximal tolerated dose of statin therapy and ezetimibe with persistently elevated LDL-C > 70 or non HDL-C > 100, the addition of PCSK9 inhibitors can be considered.

7. Current and future therapy targets for dyslipidemia ASCVD

7.1 Statins

Dyslipidemia therapy for the primary and secondary prevention of ASCVD, both current and therapies under investigation for future use, are centered on targeting LDL-C given the extensive evidence demonstrating the relationship between LDL and ASCVD, and no class of medications has been shown to be more effective at lowering LDL-C than statins, the foundation of lipid and cholesterol lowering therapy [101, 172, 173].

Statins inhibit HMG-CoA reductase, the rate-limiting enzyme in the synthetic pathway of cholesterol, resulting in lowering of tissue cholesterol, most critically intrahepatic cholesterol, and reflex increase in hepatic expression of surface LDLR and accompanying enhancement of receptor-mediated uptake of LDL and other circulating lipoproteins [172, 174]. Beyond the inhibition of hepatic cholesterol synthesis and the resulting reduction in circulating LDL, statins have demonstrated other important benefits in atherosclerotic plaque progression and the risk of acute atherothrombosis [174, 175]. Statins promote plaque stabilization by reducing inflammation and increasing collagen content in atherosclerotic plaques, slow the progression of overall plaque volume, and diminish high-risk or vulnerable plaque features [174–176].

Statin dosing intensity is categorized by expected reduction in LDL-C, with high-intensity statins typically lowering LDL-C by at least 50%, moderate-intensity statins typically lowering LDL-C by 30–49%, and low-intensity statins typically lowering LDL-C by less than 30%.

7.2 Nonstatins

There are different classes of non-statin medications used in the management of dyslipidemia, including bile acid sequestrants (cholestyramine, colestipol, and colesevelam), niacin, and fibrate, with ezetimibe and the PCSK9 inhibitors being the non-statin classes of medications that incorporated into the guidelines for dyslipidemia management in the primary and secondary prevention of ASCVD in combination therapy with statins [100].

Ezetimibe decreases small intestine cholesterol absorption by inhibiting the Niemann-Pick C1-Like 1 (NPC1L1) transporter [172, 177]. While the exact mechanisms of the effect of ezetimibe on atherosclerosis by itself are not as well defined as the effects of statins on atherosclerotic plaque progression and stabilization, the addition of ezetimibe to statins has been shown to regress plaque burden, reduce plaque volume, and promote plaque stabilization [178, 179]. PSCK9 works by interacting in with hepatic LDLR and enhancing the degradation of the receptor by hepatic lysosomes, with PSCK9 inhibitors thus mitigating the PSCK9-mediated turnover of hepatic LDLR and prolonging LDLR lifespan and uptake of circulating LDL-C [180]. PSCK9 inhibitors, namely alirocumab and evolocumab, in combination with statins have been shown to increase plaque calcification (a marker of plaque stability), and promote VSMC and collagen plaque content while simultaneously decreasing the size of the lipid necrotic core [181, 182].

7.3 New and future therapeutic targets and approaches to dyslipidemia and ASCVD

Beyond the dramatic reductions in LDL-C and mechanisms of atherosclerotic plaque stabilization and slowing of progression effected by statins, ezetimibe, and PSCK9 inhibitors and their codification in the management algorithms for dyslipidemia and ASCVD: the other inflammatory, lipoprotein, and metabolic pathways involved in the pathophysiology of atherosclerosis serve as potential targets for therapies in the primary and secondary prevention of dyslipidemia and ASCVD.

The antiatherogenic properties of HDL, both in terms of its antioxidant and cholesterol efflux capacities, have led to investigations for the therapeutic potential of reconstituted HDL and methods to improve endogenous HDL functionality [23, 183]. Apo A-1 and apolipoprotein E (Apo E) are the atheroprotective apolipoprotein components of HDL, but studies involving Apo A-1/HDL mimetic peptides transcriptional upregulators of Apo A-1 did not result in significant regression of coronary atherosclerotic lesions despite the enhanced HDL-C efflux [184]. Apo E consists of three isoforms (Apo E2, Apo E3, and Apo E4) and promotes clearance of circulating TG-rich lipoprotein remnants, cholesterol efflux from macrophages preventing foam cell formation, and diminishes expression of adhesion molecules necessary for macrophage migration into the arterial intima [184–186]. ApoE exerts additional atheroprotective functions via tampering the inflammatory response by inhibiting T cells, lipoprotein oxidation, and resulting proliferation and migration of VSMCs, suppressing platelet aggregation, and restoring endothelial function by promoting release of NO [184, 187–190]. Given ApoE diverse protective properties at various stages of the atherosclerotic thromboinflammatory process, studies investigating the potential value of reconstituted HDL with favorable ApoE content or methods to promote increased ApoE profiles among endogenous HDL can serve substantial roles for the future management of dyslipidemia and ASCVD.

Given the extensive inflammatory pathways and processes underlying the pathogenesis of atherosclerosis, considerable work has been and is currently dedicated to anti-inflammatory targets of therapy in dyslipidemia and ASCVD, with drugs in various stages of research and development. The role of lipoprotein oxidation, most significantly LDL to ox-LDL, has prompted the study of therapeutic antioxidants in the management of dyslipidemia, and has shown promising benefits in secondary prevention of ASCVD after ACS within 12 months [191, 192]. The increase of ox-LDL levels due to phospholipase A2 activity which enzymatically generate phospholipids with atherogenic modifications has led to study of the role of phospholipase 2 inhibitors in the prevention of atherosclerosis [193]. Many other inflammatory pathway targets have been investigated for the management of dyslipidemia and ASCVD including leukotriene pathway inhibitors (promote atherosclerotic plaque development and progression via chemoattraction of macrophages and other inflammatory cells and increasing endothelial permeability), chemokine CC motif ligand 2 (CCL2), also known as MCP1 (chemokine recruiter of plaque destabilizing macrophages), and blockade of potent inflammatory markers TNF and IL-1 [191, 194–196].

8. Conclusion

Atherosclerotic cardiovascular disease encompasses conditions carrying tremendous morbidity and mortality, and is the acute and chronic clinical manifestations of a progressive pathogenic process that is initiated by the inflammatory responses to dyslipidemia. The diverse metabolic and immune mechanisms at play in the thrombo-inflammatory pathophysiology of atherosclerosis are driven by disruptions in the body's native metabolism of cholesterol, triglycerides, and lipoproteins, with comorbid conditions and risk factors such as smoking, hypertension, and obesity promoting critical changes in cholesterol and lipoproteins that initiate a vicious cycle of lipoprotein accumulation, foam cell formation, and inflammatory reaction. The fact that so many immune cell lines and metabolic factors play important roles in the development of atherosclerosis serves as a pool of current and potential future targets for therapies in the primary and secondary prevention of dyslipidemia and ASCVD.

Author details

Perry Wengrofsky[1], Justin Lee[2] and Amgad N. Makaryus[3,4*]

1 Department of Internal Medicine, State University of New York, Downstate Medical Center, Brooklyn, NY, USA

2 Division of Cardiovascular Disease, Department of Medicine, State University of New York, Downstate Medical Center, Brooklyn, NY, USA

3 Department of Cardiology, Nassau University Medical Center, East Meadow, NY, USA

4 Donald and Barbara Zucker School of Medicine at Hofstra/Northwell, Hempstead, NY, USA

*Address all correspondence to: amakaryu@numc.edu

References

[1] Wu MY, Li CK, Hou MF, Chu PY. New insights into the role of inflammation in the pathogenesis of atherosclerosis. International Journal of Molecular Sciences. 2017;**18**(10): 2034, 1-18

[2] Rafieian-Kopaei M, Setorki M, Doudi M, Baradaran A, Nasri H. Atherosclerosis: Process, indicators, risk factors and new hopes. International Journal of Preventive Medicine. 2014;**5**(8):927-946

[3] Rader DJ, Pure E. Lipoproteins, macrophage function, and atherosclerosis: Beyond the foam cell. Cell Metabolism. 2005;**1**(4):223-230

[4] Helkin A, Stein JS, Lin S, et al. Dyslipidemia. Part I—Review of lipid metabolism and vascular cell physiology. Vascular and Endovascular Surgery. 2016;**50**(2):107-118

[5] Ference BA, Ginsberg HN, Graham I, et al. Low-density lipoproteins cause atherosclerotic cardiovascular disease. 1. Evidence from genetic, epidemiologic, and clinical studies. A consensus statement from the european atherosclerosis society consensus panel. European Heart Journal. 2017;**38**:2459-2472

[6] Feingold KR, Grunfeld C. Introduction to lipids and lipoproteins. In: De Groot LJ, Chrousos G, Dungan K, et al., editors. Endotext [Internet]. South Darmouth (MA): MDText.com, Inc.; 2000. Available from: https://www.ncbi.nlm.nih.gov/books/NBK305896/ [Accessed: Feb 2, 2018]

[7] Chan DC, Watts GF. Apolipoproteins as markers and managers of coronary risk. QJM: An International Journal of Medicine. 2006;**99**(5):277-287

[8] Laler PR, Akinkuolie AO, Chu AY, et al. Atherogenic lipoprotein determinants of cardiovascular disease and residual risk among individuals with low low-density lipoprotein cholesterol. Journal of the American Heart Association. 2017;**6**(7): e005549, 1-17

[9] Navab M, Reddy ST, Van Lenten BJ, Fogelman AM. HDL and cardiovascular disease: Atherogenic and atheroprotective mechanisms. Nature. 2011;**8**:222-232

[10] Tomkin GH, Owens D. The chylomicron: Relationship to atherosclerosis. International Journal of Vascular Medicine. 2012;**2012**:784536

[11] Wilhelm MG, Cooper AD. Induction of atherosclerosis by human chylomicron remnants. Journal of Atherosclerosis and Thrombosis. 2003;**10**(3):132-139

[12] Nakajima K, Nagamine T, Fujita MQ, et al. Apolipoprotein B-48: A unique marker of chylomicron metabolism. Advances in Clinical Chemistry. 2014;**64**:117-177

[13] Kei AA, Filippatos TD, Tsimihodimos V, Elisaf MS. A review of the role of apolioprotein C-II in lipoprotein metabolism and cardiovascular disease. Metabolism. 2012;**61**(7):906-921

[14] Olofsson SO, Boren J. Apolipoprotein B: A clinically important apolipoprotein which assembles atherogenic lipoproteins and prompts the development of atherosclerosis. Journal of Internal Medicine. 2005;**258**:395-410

[15] Nordestgaard BG, Tybjaerg-Hansen A. IDL, VLDL, chylomicrons and atherosclerosis. European Journal of Epidemiology. 1992;**8**(Suppl 1):92-98

[16] Carmena R, Duriez P, Fruchart JC. Atherogenic lipoprotein particles

in atherosclerosis. Circulation. 2004;**109**(Suppl III):III-2-III-7

[17] Ivanova EA, Myasoedova VA, Melnichenko AA, et al. Small dense low-density lipoprotein as biomarker for atherosclerotic diseases. Oxidative Medicine and Cellular Longevity. 2017;**2017**:1273042

[18] Goldstein JL, Brown MS. The LDL receptor. Arteriosclerosis, Thrombosis, and Vascular Biology. 2009;**29**(4):431-438

[19] Horton JD, Cohen JC, Hobbs HH. Molecular biology of PCSK9: Its role in LDL metabolism. Trends in Biochemical Sciences. 2007;**32**(2):71-77

[20] Suma V, Sanyal S, Thakur A, Makaryus A, Hecht H. Abstract 1185: Changes in small dense LDL particle distrbution with addition of niacin to a statin regimen. Do the lipid sub-fractions change to a less atherogenic pattern? Circulation. 2008;**118**:S_1080-S_1081

[21] Bandeali S, Farmer J. High-density lipoprotein and atherosclerosis: The role of antioxidant activity. Current Atherosclerosis Reports. 2012;**14**:101-107

[22] Rye KA, Barter PJ. Cardioprotective functions of HDLs. Journal of Lipid Research. 2014;**55**(2):168-179

[23] Rosenson RS, Brewer BB Jr, Ansell BJ, et al. Dysfunctional HDL and atherosclerotic cardiovascular disease. Nature. 2016;**13**:48-60

[24] Nordestgaard BG, Chapman MJ, Ray K, et al. Lipoprotein(a) as a cardiovascular risk factor: Current status. European Heart Journal. 2010;**31**:2844-2853

[25] Koschinsky ML. Lipoprotein(a) and atherosclerosis. New perspectives on the mechanism of action of an enigmatic lipoprotein. Current Atherosclerosis Reports. 2005;**7**:389-395

[26] Nielsen LB. Atherogenecity of lipoprotein(a) and oxidized low density lipoprotein: Insight from in vivo studeis of arterial wall influx. Degradation and Efflux. Atheroscler. 1999;**143**:229-243

[27] Feric NT, Boffa MB, Johnston SM, Koschinsky ML. Apolipoprotein(a) inhibits the conversion of Glu-plasminogen to Lys-plasminogen: A novel mechanism for lipoprotein(a)-mediated inhibition of plasminogen activation. Journal of Thrombosis and Haemostasis. 2008;**6**:2113-2120

[28] Gimbrone MA Jr, Garcia-Cardena G. Endothelial cell dysfunction and the pathobiology of atherosclerosis. Circulation Research. 2016;**118**(4):620-636

[29] Forstermann U, Xia N, Li H. Roles of vascular oxidative stress and nitric oxide in the pathogenesis of atherosclerosis. Circulation Research. 2017;**120**:713-735

[30] Pernow J, Shemyakin A, Bohm F. New perspectives on endothelin-1 in atherosclerosis and diabetes mellitus. Life Sciences. 2012;**91**(13-14):507-516

[31] Li YS, Haga JH, Chien S. Molecular basis of the effects of shear stress on vascular endothelial cells. Journal of Biomechanics. 2005;**38**(10):1949-1971

[32] Tabas I, Garcia-Cardena G, Owens GK. Recent insights into the cellular biology of atherosclerosis. Journal of Cell Biology. 2015;**209**(1):13-22

[33] Mitra R, O'Neil GL, Harding IC, et al. Glycocalyx in atherosclerosis-relevant endothelium function as a therapeutic target. Current Atherosclerosis Reports. 2017;**19**(12):63

[34] Linton MF, Yancey PG, Davies SS, et al. The role of lipids and lipoproteins in atherosclerosis. In: De Groot LJ,

Chrousos G, Dungan K, et al., editors. WEndotext [Internet]. South Dartmouth (MA): MDText.com, Inc.; 2000. Available from: https://www.ncbi.nlm.nih.gov/books/NBK343489/ [Accessed: Dec 24, 2015]

[35] Tabas I, Williams KJ, Boren J. Subendothelial lipoprotein retention as the initiating process in atherosclerosis. Update and therapeutic implications. Circulation. 2007;**116**(16):1832-1844

[36] Milstone DS, Ilyama M, Chen M, et al. Differential role of an NF- κB transcriptional response element in endothelial versus intimal cell VCAM-1 expression. Circulation Research. 2015;**117**:166-177

[37] Ramji DP, Davies TS. Cytokines in atherosclerosis: Key players in all stages of disease and promising therapeutic targets. Cytokine & Growth Factor Reviews. 2015;**26**(6):673-685

[38] Boullier A, Bird DA, Chang MK, et al. Scavenger receptors, oxidized LDL, and atherosclerosis. Annals of the New York Academy of Sciences. 2001;**947**:214-222

[39] Gistera A, Hansson GK. The immunology of atherosclerosis. Nature. 2017;**13**:368-380

[40] Miller YI, Choi SH, Fang L, Tsimikas S. Lipoprotein modification and macrophage uptake: Role of pathologic cholesterol transport in atherogenesis. Sub-Cellular Biochemistry. 2010;**51**:229-251

[41] Bleda S, de Haro K, Varela C, et al. Elevated levels of triglycerides and VLDL-cholesterol provoke activation of NLRP1 inflammasone in endothelial cells. International Journal of Cardiology. 2016;**220**:52-55

[42] Vaughan DE. PAI-1 and atherothrombosis. Journal of Thrombosis and Haemostasis. 2005;**3**:1879-1883

[43] Riches K, Porter KE. Lipoprotein(a): Cellular effects and molecular mechanisms. Cholesterol. 2012;**2012**:923289

[44] Lara-Guzman OJ, Gil-Izquierdo A, Medina S, et al. Oxidized LDL triggers changes in oxidative stress and inflammatory biomarkers in human macrophages. Redox Biology. 2018;**15**:1-11

[45] Zernecke A. Dendritic cells in atherosclerosis: Evidence in mice and humans. Arteriosclerosis, Thrombosis, and Vascular Biology. 2015;**35**:763-770

[46] Gronberg C, Nilsson J, Wigren M. Recent advances on CD4+ T cells in atherosclerosis and its implications for therapy. European Journal of Pharmacology. 2017;**816**:58-66

[47] van Duijn J, Kuiper J, Slutter B. The many faces of CD8+ T cells in atherosclerosis. Current Opinion in Lipidology. 2018;**28**(5):411-416

[48] Tabas I, Lichtman AH. Monocyte-macrophages and T cells in atherosclerosis. Immunity. 2017;**74**(4):621-634

[49] Decano JL, Aikawa M. Dynamic macrophages: Understanding mechanisms of activation as guide to therapy for atherosclerotic vascular disease. Frontiers in Cardiovascular Medicine. 2018;**5**:97

[50] Tabas I. Macrophage death and defective inflammation resolution in atherosclerosis. Nature Reviews Immunology. 2010;**10**:36-46

[51] Subramanian M, Tabas I. Dendritic cells in atherosclerosis. Seminars in Immunopathology. 2014;**36**(1):93-102

[52] Bennet MR, Sinha S, Owens GK. Vascular smooth muscle cells in

atherosclerosis. Circulation Research. 2016;**118**(4):692-702

[53] Wang J, Uryga AK, Reinhold J, et al. Vascular smooth muscle cell senescence promotes atherosclerosis and features of plaque vulnerability. Atherosclerosis. 2015;**132**(20):1909-1919

[54] Gomez D, Owens GK. Smooth muscle cell phenotypic switching in atherosclerosis. Cardiovascular Research. 2012;**95**(2):156-164

[55] Ponticos M, Smith BD. Extracellular matrix synthesis in vascular disease. hypertension, and atherosclerosis. Journal of Biomedical Research. 2014;**28**(1):25-39

[56] Toma I, McCaffrey TA. Transforming growth factor-β and atherosclerosis: Interwoven atherogenic and atheroprotective aspects. Cell and Tissue Research. 2012;**347**(1):155-175

[57] Tedgui A, Mallat Z. Cytokines in atherosclerosis: Pathogenic and regulatory pathways. Physiological Reviews. 2006;**86**:515-581

[58] Brites F, Martin M, Guillas I, Kontush A. Antioxidative activity of high-density lipoprotein (HDL): Mechanistic insights into potential clinical benefit. BBA Clinical. 2017;**8**:66-77

[59] Singh K, Singh R, Chandra S, Tyagi S. Paraoxonase-1 is a better indicator than HDL of atherosclerosis—A pilot study in North Indian population. Diabetes and Metabolic Syndrome: Clinical Research and Reviews. 2018;**12**(3):275-268

[60] Peng ZY, Zhao SP, He BM, et al. Protective effect of HDL on endothelial NO production: The role of DDAH/ADMA pathway. Molecular and Cellular Biochemistry. 2011;**351**(1-2):243-249

[61] Tran-Dinh A, Diallo D, Delbosc S, et al. HDL and endothelial protection. British Journal of Pharmacology. 2013;**169**(3):493-511

[62] Barter PJ, Nicholls S, Rye KA, et al. Antiinflammatory properties of HDL. Circulation Research. 2004;**95**:764-772

[63] Ganjali S, Gotto AM Jr, Ruscica M, et al. Monocyte-to-HDL-cholesterol ratio as a prognostic marker in cardiovascular disease. Journal of Cellular Physiology. 2018;**233**(12):9237-9246

[64] van der Stoep M, Korporaai SJ, Van Eck M. High-density lipoprotein as a modulator of platelet and coagulation responses. Cardiovascular Research. 2014;**103**(3):362-371

[65] Phillips MC. Molecular mechanisms of cellular cholesterol efflux. The Journal of Biological Chemistry. 2014;**289**(35):24020-24029

[66] Yancey PG, Bortnick AE, Kellner-Weibel G, et al. Importance of different pathways of cellular cholesterol efflux. Arteriosclerosis, Thrombosis, and Vascular Biology. 2003;**23**(5):712-719

[67] Lee MK, Moore XL, Fu Y, et al. High-density lipoprotein inhibits human M1 macorphage polarization through redistribution of caveolin-1. British Journal of Pharmacology. 2016;**173**(4):741-751

[68] Sanson M, Distel E, Fisher EA. HDL induces the expression of the M2 macrophage markers arginase 1 and fizz-1 in a STAT6-depedent process. PLoS One. 2013;**8**(8):e74676

[69] Terasaka N, Wang N, Yvan-Charvet L, Tall AR. High-density lipoprotein protects macrophages from oxidized low-density lipoprotein-induced apoptosis by promoting efflux of 7-ketocholesterol via ABCG1. Proceedings of the National Academy

of Sciences of the United States of America. 2007;**104**(38):15093-15098

[70] Insull W Jr. The pathology of atherosclerosis. Plaque development and plaque responses to medical treatment. The American Journal of Medicine. 2009;**122**(1):S3-S14

[71] Sakakura K, Nakano M, Otsuka F, et al. Pathophysiology of atherosclerosis plaque progression. Heart, Lung Circulation. 2013;**22**(6):399-411

[72] Martinet W, Schrijvers DM, De Meyer GRY. Necrotic cell death in atherosclerosis. Basic Research in Cardiology. 2011;**106**:749-760

[73] Kojima Y, Weissman IL, Leeper NJ. The role of efferocytosis in atherosclerosis. Circulation. 2017;**135**:476-489

[74] Weinert S, Poitz DM, Auffermann-Gretzinger S, et al. The lysosomal transfer of LDL/cholesterol from macrophages into vascular smooth muscle cells induces their phenotypic alteration. Cardiovascular Research. 2013;**97**(3):544-542

[75] Singh RB, Mengi SA, Xu YJ, et al. Pathogenesis of atherosclerosis: A multifactorial process. Experimental and Clinical Cardiology. 2002;7(1):40-53

[76] Matsuo Y, Takumi T, Matthew V, et al. Plaque characteristics and arterial remodeling in coronary and peripheral arterial systems. Atherosclerosis. 2012;**223**(2):365-371

[77] van der Wal AC, Becker AE. Atherosclerotic plaque rupture—Pathologic basis of plaque stability and instability. Cardiovascular Research. 1999;**41**(2):334-344

[78] Halvorsen B, Otterdal K, Dahl TB, et al. Atherosclerotic plaque stability—What determines the fate of a plaque? Progress in Cardiovascular Diseases. 2008;**51**(3):183-194

[79] Osborn EA, Jaffer FA. Imaging atherosclerosis and risk of plaque rupture. Current Atherosclerosis Reports. 2013;**15**(10):359

[80] Nadkarni SK, Bilenca A, Bouma BE, Tearney GJ. Measurement of fibrous cap thickness in athersclerotic plaques by spatiotemporal analysis of laser speckle images. Journal of Biomedical Optics. 2006;**11**(2):021006

[81] Newby AC. Metalloproteinases and vulnerable atherosclerotic plaques. Trends in Cardiovascular Medicine. 2007;**17**(8):253-258

[82] Johnson JL. Metalloproteinases in atherosclerosis. European Journal of Pharmacology. 2017;**816**:93-106

[83] Ruddy JM, Ikonomdis JS, Jones JA. Multidimensional contribution of matrix metalloproteinases to atherosclerotic plaque vulnerability: Multiple mechanisms of inhibition to promote stability. Journal of Vascular Research. 2015;**53**:1-16

[84] Clarke MC, Figg N, Maguire JJ, et al. Apoptosis of vascular smooth muscle cells induces features of plaque vulnerability in atherosclerosis. Nature Medicine. 2006;**12**:1075-1080

[85] Rohm I, Atiskova Y, Drobnik S, et al. Decreased regulatory T cells in vulnerable atherosclerotic lesions: Imbalance between pro- and anti-inflammatory cells in atherosclerosis. Mediators of Inflammation. 2015;**2015**:364710

[86] Ammirati E, Moroni F, Magnoni M, Camici PG. The role of T and B cells in human atherosclerosis and atherothrombosis. Clinical and Experimental Immunology. 2015;**179**(2):173-187

[87] Lafont A. Basic aspects of plaque vulnerability. Heart. 2003;**89**(10): 1262-1267

[88] Badimon L, Pardo T, Vilahur G. Atherosclerosis, platelets and thrombosis in acute ischaemic heart disease. European Heart Journal Acute Cardiovascular Care. 2012;**1**(1):60-74

[89] Sato Y, Hatakeyama K, Yamashita A, et al. Proportion of fibrin and platelets differs in thrombi on ruptured and eroded coronary atherosclerotic plaques in humans. Heart. 2005;**91**:526-530

[90] Olie RH, van der Meijden PEJ, ten Cate H. The coagulation system in atherothrombosis: Implications for new therapeutic strategies. Research and Practice in Thrombosis and Haemostasis. 2018;**2**:188-198

[91] Wu MD, Atkinson TM, Lindner JR. Platelets and von Willebrand factor in atherogenesis. Blood. 2017;**129**(11):1415-1419

[92] Guo S, Shen S, Wang J, et al. Detection of high-risk atherosclerotic plaques with ultrasound molecular imaging of glycoprotein IIb/IIIa receptor on activated platelets. Theranostics. 2015;**5**(2):418-430

[93] Bogousslavsky J. Benefit of ADP receptor antagonists in atherothrombotic patients: New evidence. Cerebrovascular Diseases. 2011;**11**(Suppl 2):5-10

[94] Moons AHM, Levi M, Peters RJG. Tissue factor and coronary artery disease. Cardiovascular Research. 2002;**53**(2):313-325

[95] Tatsumi K, Machman N. Tissue factor and atherothrombosis. Journal of Atherosclerosis and Thrombosis. 2015;**22**(6):543-549

[96] Leonardi S, Becker RC. PAR-1 inhibitors: A novel class of antiplatelet agents for the treatment of patients with atherothrombosis. Handbook of Experimental Pharmacology. 2012;**210**:239-260

[97] van Montfoort ML, Kuijpers MJE, Knaup VL, et al. Factor XI regulates pathological thrombus formation on acutely ruptured atherosclerotic plaques. Arteriosclerosis, Thrombosis, and Vascular Biology. 2014;**34**:1668-1673

[98] Uchida Y, Uchida Y, Sakurai T, et al. Characterization of coronary fibrin thrombus in patients with acute coronary syndrome using dye-staining angioscopy. Arteriosclerosis, Thrombosis, and Vascular Biology. 2011;**31**:1452-1460

[99] Niesten JM, van der Schaaf IC, van Dam L, et al. Histopathologic composition of cerebral thrombi of acute stroke patients is correlated with stroke subtype and thrombus attenuation. PLoS One. 2014;**9**(2):e88882

[100] Anderson TJ, Gregoire J, Pearson GJ, et al. 2016 Canadian Cardiovascular Society Guidelines for the management of dyslipidemia for the prevention of cardiovascular disease in the adult. The Canadian Journal of Cardiology. 2016;**32**(11):1263-1282

[101] Grundy SM, Stone NJ, Bailey AL, et al. 2018 AHA/ACC/AACVPR/AAPA/ABC/ACPM/ADA/AGS/APhA/ASPC/NLA/PCNA Guideline on the management of blood cholesterol. Journal of the American College of Cardiology. 2018. pii: S0735-1097(18)39033-8

[102] Catapano AL, Graham I, De Backer G, et al. 2016 ESC/EAS Guidelines for the management of dyslipidaemias. European Heart Journal. 2016;**37**(39):2999-3058

[103] Gerhard-Herman MD, Gornik HL, Barret C, et al. 2016 AHA/ACC

Guideline on the management of patients with lower extremity peripheral artery disease. Journal of the American College of Cardiology. 2017;**69**(11):e71-e126

[104] Levine GN, Bates ER, Bittl JA, et al. 2016 ACC/AHA Guideline focused update on duration of dual antiplatelet therapy in patients with coronary artery disease. Journal of the American College of Cardiology. 2016;**68**(10):1082-1115

[105] Levine GN, Bates ER, Blankenship JC, et al. 2015 ACC/AHA/SCAI focused update on primary percutaneous coronary intervention for patients with ST-elevation myocardial infarction. Journal of the American College of Cardiology. 2016;**67**(10):1235-1250

[106] Amsterdam EA, Wenger NK, Brindis RG, et al. 2014 AHA/ACC Guideline for the management of patients with non-ST-elevation acute coronary syndromes. Journal of the American College of Cardiology. 2014;**64**(24):e139-e228

[107] Fihn SD, Gardin JM, Abrams J, et al. 2012 ACC/AHA/ACP/AATS/PCNA/SCAI/STS Guideline for the diagnosis and management of patients with stable ischemic heart disease. Journal of the American College of Cardiology. 2012;**60**(24):e44-e164

[108] Anderson JL, Halperin JL, Albert N, et al. Management of patients with peripheral artery disease (compilation of 2005 and 2011 ACCF/AHA Guideline recommendations). Journal of the American College of Cardiology. 2013;**61**(14):1555-1570

[109] O'Gara PT, Kushner FG, Ascheim DD, et al. 2013 ACCF/AHA Guideline for the management of ST-elevation myocardial infarction. Journal of the American College of Cardiology. 2013;**61**(4):e78-e140

[110] Smith SC Jr, Benjamin EJ, Bonow RO, et al. AHA/ACCF secondary prevention and risk reduction therapy for patients with coronary and other atherosclerotic vascular disease: 2011 update. A guideline from the American Heart Association and American College of Cardiology Foundation endorsed by the World Heart Federation and the Preventive Cardiovascular Nurses Association. Journal of the American College of Cardiology. 2011;**58**(23):2432-2446

[111] Brott TG, Halperin JL, Abbara S, et al. 2011 ASA/ACCF/AHA/AANN/AANS/ACR/ASNR/CNS/SAIP/SCAI/SIR/SNIS/SVM/SVS Guideline on the management of patients with extracranial carotid and vertebral artery disease. Journal of the American College of Cardiology. 2011;**57**(8):e16-e94

[112] Powers WJ, Rabinstein AA, Ackerson T, et al. 2018 Guidelines for the early management of patients with acute ischemic stroke: A guideline for healthcare professionals from the American Heart Association/American Stroke Association. Stroke. 2018;**49**:e46-e99

[113] Committee W, Das SR, Everett BM, Birtcher KK, et al. ACC expert consensus decision pathway on novel therapies for cardiovascular risk reduction in patients with type 2 diabetes and atherosclerotic cardiovascular disease. Journal of the American College of Cardiology. 2018;**2018**:25566. DOI: 10.1016/j.jacc.2018.09.020

[114] Llyod-Jones DM, Morris PB, Ballantyne CM, et al. 2017 Focused update on the 2016 ACC expert consensus decision pathway on the role of non-statin therapies for LDL-cholesterol lowering in the management of atherosclerotic cardiovascular disease risk. Journal of the American College of Cardiology. 2017;**70**(14):1785-1822

[115] Thygesen K, Alpert JS, Jaffe AS, et al. Fourth universal definition of

myocardial infarction. Journal of the American College of Cardiology. 2018;**2018**:25285. DOI: 10.1016/j.jacc.2018.08.1038

[116] Ford TJ, Corcoran D, Berry C, et al. Stable coronary syndromes: Pathophysiology, diagnostic advances and therapeutic need. Heart. 2017;**0**:1-9

[117] Ohman EM. Clinical practice. Chronic stable angina. New England Journal of Medicine. 2016;**374**(12):1167-1176

[118] Greenland P, Blaha M, Budoff MJ, Erbel R, Watson KE. Coronary calcium score and cardiovascular risk. Journal of the American College of Cardiology. 2018;**72**(4):4343-4447

[119] Eisen A, Giugliano RP, Braunwald E. Updates on acute coronary syndrome: A review. JAMA Cardiology. 2016;**1**(6):718-730

[120] Trzeciak P, Gierlotka M, Gasior M, et al. In-hospital and 12-month outcomes after acute coronary syndrome treatment in patients aged <40 years of age (from the Polish Registry of Acute Coronary Syndromes). American Journal of Cardiology. 2014;**114**(2):175-180

[121] Puymirat E, Simon T, Cayla G, et al. Acute myocardial infarction: Changes in patient characteristics, management, and 6-month outcomes over a period of 20 years in the FAST-MI program (French Registry of Acute ST-Elevation or Non-ST-Elevation Myocardial Infarction 1995 to 2015). Circulation. 2017;**136**(20):1908-1919

[122] Lippi G, Sanchis-Gomar F, Cervellin G. Cardiac troponins and mortality in type 1 and 2 myocardial infarction. Clinical Chemistry and Laboratory Medicine. 2017;**55**(2):181-188

[123] Jangaard N, Sarkisian L, Saaby L, et al. Incidence, frequency, and clinical characteristics of type 3 myocardial infarction in clinical practice. American Journal of Medicine. 2017;**130**(7):862.e9-e862.e14

[124] Cediel G, Sandoval Y, Sexter A, et al. Risk estimation in type 2 myocardial infarction and myocardial injury: The TARRACO risk score. American Journal of Medicine. 2019;**132**(2):217-226

[125] Hills LD, Smith PK, Anderson JL, et al. 2011 ACCF/AGA Guideline for coronary artery bypass graft surgery. Journal of the American College of Cardiology. 2011;**58**(24):e123-e210

[126] Levine GN, Bates ER, Blankenship JC, et al. 2011 ACCF/AHA/SCAI Guideline for percutaneous coronary intervention. Journal of the American College of Cardiology. 2011;**58**(24):e44-e122

[127] Bashore TM, Balter S, Barac A, et al. 2012 American College of Cardiology Foundation/society for cardiovascular angiography and interventions expert consensus document on cardiac catheterization laboratory standards update. Journal of the American College of Cardiology. 2012;**59**(24):2221-2305

[128] Banerjee C, Chimowitz MI. Stroke caused by atherosclerosis of the major intracranial arteries. Circulation Research. 2017;**120**:502-513

[129] An SJ, Kim TJ, Yoon BW. Epidemiology, risk factors, and clinical features of intracerebral hemorrhage: An update. Journal of Stroke. 2017;**19**(1):3-10

[130] Woo D, Haverbusch M, Sekar P, et al. Effect of untreated hypertension on hemorrhagic stroke. Stroke. 2004;**35**:1703-1708

[131] Prabhakaran S, Ruff I, Bernstein RA. Acute stroke intervention: A systematic review. Journal of the American Medical Association. 2015;**313**(14):1451-1462

[132] Ceornodolea AD, Bal R, Severens JL. Epidemiology and management of atrial fibrillation and stroke: Review of data from four European countries. Stroke Research and Treatment. 2017;**2017**:8593207

[133] Smith EE, Kent DM, Bulsara KR, et al. Accuracy of prediction instruments for diagnosing large vessel occlusion in individuals with suspected stroke: A systematic review for the 2018 Guidelines for the early management of patients with acute ischemic stroke. Stroke. 2018;**49**:e111-e122

[134] Meschia JF, Bushnell C, Boden-Albala B, et al. Guidelines for the primary prevention of stroke: A statement for healthcare professionals from the American Heart Association/ American Stroke Association. Stroke. 2014;**45**:3754-3832

[135] Hiatt WR, Goldstone J, Smith SC Jr, et al. Atherosclerotic peripheral vascular disease symposium II: Nomenclature for vascular diseases. Circulation. 2008;**118**:2826-2829

[136] Kullo IJ, Rooke TW. Clinical practice. Peripheral artery disease. New England Journal of Medicine. 2016;**374**(9):861-871

[137] Creager MA, Kaufman JA, Conte MS. Clinical practice. Acute limb ischemia. New England Journal of Medicine. 2012;**366**:2198-2206

[138] Enezate TH, Omran J, Mahmud E, et al. Endovascular versus surgical treatment for acute limb ischemia: A systematic review and meta-analysis of clinical trials. Cardiovascular Diagnosis and Therapy. 2017;7(3):264-271

[139] Theodoridis PG, Davos CH, Dodos I, et al. Thrombolysis in acute lower limb ischemia. Review of the current literature. Annals of Vascular Surgery. 2018;**52**:255-262

[140] Kinlay SK. Management of critical limb ischemia. Circulation. Cardiovascular Interventions. 2016;**9**(2):e001946

[141] Fabiani I, Calogero E, Pugliese NR, et al. Critical limb ischemia: A practical up-to-date review. Angiology. 2018;**69**(6):465-474

[142] Teraa M, Conte MS, Moll FL, Verhaar MC. Critical limb ischemia: Current trends and future directions. Journal of the American Heart Association. 2016;**5**:e002938

[143] Pollak AW, Norton P, Kramer CM. Multimodality imaging of lower extremity peripheral arterial disease: Current role and future directions. Circulation. Cardiovascular Imaging. 2012;**5**(6):797-807

[144] Shishehbor MH, White CJ, Gray BH, et al. Critical limb ischemia: An expert statement. Journal of the American College of Cardiology. 2016;**68**(16):2002-2015

[145] Walker TG. Acute limb ischemia. Techniques in Vascular and Interventional Radiology. 2009;**12**(2):117-129

[146] Weber BR, Dieter RS. Renal artery stenosis: Epidemiology and treatment. Iternational Journal of Nephrology and Renovascular Disease An international. 2014;7:169-181

[147] Gottam N, Nanjundappa A, Dieter RS. Renal artery stenosis: Pathophysiology and treatment. Expert Review of Cardiovascular Therapy. 2009;7(11):1413-1420

[148] Garovic VD, Textor SC. Renovascular hypertension and

ischemic nephropathy. Circulation. 2005;**112**:1362-1374

[149] AbuRahma AF, Yacoub M. Renal imaging: Duplex ultrasound, computed tomography angiography, magnestic resonance angiography, and angiography. Seminars in Vascular Surgery. 2013;**26**(4):134-143

[150] Bavishi C, de Leeuw PW, Messerli FH. Atherosclerotic renal artery stenosis and hypertension: Pragmatism, pitfalls, and perspectives. American Journal of Medicine. 2016;**129**(6):635.e5-635.e14

[151] Tafur JD, White CJ. Renal artery stenosis: When to revascularize in 2017. Current Problems in Cardiology. 2017;**42**(4):110-135

[152] Hohenwalter EJ. Chronic mesenteric ischemia: Diagnosis and treatment. Seminars in Interventional Radiology. 2009;**26**(4):345-351

[153] Zettervall SL, Lo RC, Soden PA, et al. Trends in treatment and mortality for mesenteric ischemia in the United States from 2000-2012. Annals of Vascular Surgery. 2017;**42**:111-119

[154] Bala M, Kashuk J, Moore EE, et al. Acute mesenteric ischemia: Guidelines of the world society of emergency surgery. World Journal of Emergency Surgery. 2017;**12**:38

[155] Dhatt HS, Behr SC, Miracle A, Wang ZJ, Yeh BM. Radiological evaluation of bowel ischemia. Radiologic Clinics of North America. 2015;**53**(6):1241-1254

[156] Tilsed JVT, Casamassima A, Kurihara H, et al. ESTES Guidelines: Acute mesenteric ischemia. European Journal of Trauma and Emergency Surgery. 2016;**42**:253-270

[157] Toghill BJ, Saratzis A, Brown MJ. Abdominal Aortic Aneurysm—An independent disease to atherosclerosis? Cardiovascular Pathology. 2017;**27**:71-75

[158] Hong H, Yang Y, Liu B, Cai W. Imaging of abdominal aortic aneurysm: The present and the future. Current Vascular Pharmacology. 2010;**8**(6):808-819

[159] Goldstein JL, Brown MS. A century of cholesterol and coronaries: From plaques to genes to statins. Cell. 2015;**161**(1):161-172

[160] Perak AM, Ning H, de Ferranti SD, et al. Long-term risk of atherosclerotic cardiovascular disease in US adults with the familial hypercholesterolemia phenotype. Circulation. 2016;**134**(1):9-19

[161] Ogura M, Hori M, Harada-Shiba M. Association between cholesterol efflux capacity and atherosclerotic cardiovascular disease in patients with familial hypercholesterolemia. Arteriosclerosis, Thrombosis, and Vascular Biology. 2016;**36**(1):181-188

[162] Emerging Risk Factors Collaboration, Di Angelantonio E, Gao P, et al. Lipid-related markers and cardiovascular disease prediciton. Journal of the American Medical Association. 2012;**307**:2499-2506

[163] Cholesterol Treatment Trialists' (CTT) Collaboration, Baigent C, Blackwell L, et al. Efficacy and safety of more intensive lowering of LDL cholesterol: A meta-analysis of data from 170,000 participants in 26 randomized trials. Lancet. 2010;**376**:1670-1681

[164] Nissen SE, Nicholls SJ, Sipahi I, et al. Effect of very high-intensity statin therapy on regression of coronary atherosclerosis: The ASTEROID trial. Journal of the American Medical Association. 2006;**295**:1556-1565

[165] Egede LE, Zheng D. Modifiable cardiovascular risk factors in adults

with diabetes: Prevalence and missed opportunities for physician counseling. Archives of Internal Medicine. 2002;**162**(4):427-433

[166] Huma S, Tariq R, Amin F, Mahmood KJ. Modifiable and non-modifiable predisposing risk factors of myocardial infarction—A review. Journal of Pharmaceutical Sciences and Research. 2012;**4**(1):1649-1653

[167] Yang EH. Lipid management guidelines. Medscape Cardiology. 2018. Available form: https://emedicine.medscape.com/article/2500032-overview [Accessed January 11, 2019]

[168] Zeadin MG, Petlura CI, Werstuck GH. Molecular mechanisms linking diabetes to the accelerated development of atherosclerosis. Canadian Journal of Diabetes. 2013;**37**(5):345-350

[169] Shah MS, Brownlee M. Molecular and cellular mechanisms of cardiovascular disorders in diabetes. Circulation Research. 2016;**118**(11):1808-1829

[170] Kanter JE, Kramer F, Barnhart S, et al. Diabetes promotes an inflammatory macrophage phenotype and atherosclerosis through Acyl-CoA sythetase 1. Proceedings of the National Academy of Sciences of the United States of America. 2012;**109**(12):E715-E724

[171] Virmani R, Burke AP, Kolodgie F. Morphological characteristics of coronary atherosclerosis in diabetes mellitus. Canadian Journal of Cardiology. 2006;**22**(Suppl B):81B-84B

[172] Wadhera RK, Steen DL, Khan I, et al. A review of low-density lipoprotein cholesterol, treatment strategies, and its impact on cardiovascular disease morbidity and mortality. Journal of Clinical Lipidology. 2016;**10**(3):472-489

[173] Koskinas KC, Siontis GCM, Piccolo R, et al. Effect of statins and non-statin LDL-lowering medications on cardiovascular outcomes in secondary prevention: A meta-analysis of randomized trials. European Heart Journal. 2018;**39**(14):1172-1180

[174] Satoh M, Takahashi Y, Tabuchi T, et al. Cellular and molecular mechanisms of satins: An update on pleiotropic effects. Clinical Science (London, England). 2015;**129**(2):93-105

[175] Lee SE, Chang HJ, Sung JM, et al. Effects on statins on coronary atherosclerotic plaques: The PARADIGM study. JACC: Cardiovascular Imaging. 2018;**11**(10):1475-1484

[176] Yla-Herttula S, Bentzon JF, Daemen M, et al. Stabilization of atherosclerotic plaques: An update. European Heart Journal. 2013;**34**:3251-3258

[177] Vavlukis M, Vavlukis A. Adding ezetimibe to statin therapy: Latest evidence and clinical implications. Drugs in Context. 2018;**7**:212534

[178] Bogiatzi C, Spence JD. Ezetimibe and regression of carotid atherosclerosis: Importance of measuring plaque burden. Stroke. 2012;**43**(4):1153-1155

[179] Ueda Y, Hiro T, Hirayama A, et al. Effect of ezetimibe on stabilization and regression of intracoronary plaque—The ZIPANGU study. Circulation Journal. 2017;**81**(11):1611-1619

[180] Shapiro MD, Fazio S. PSCK9 and atherosclerosis—Lipids and beyond. Journal of Atherosclerosis and Thrombosis. 2017;**24**:462-472

[181] Ikegami Y, Inoue I, Inoue K, et al. The annual rate of coronary artery calcification with combination

therapy with a PSCK9 inhibitor and a statin is lower than that with statin monotherapy. NPJ Aging and Mechanisms of Disease. 2018;**4**:7

[182] Kuhnast S, van der Hoorn JWA, Pieterman EJ, et al. Alirocumab inhibits atherosclerosis, improves the plaque morphology, and enhances the effects of a statin. Journal of Lipid Research. 2014;**55**(10):2103-2112

[183] Lacy M, Atzler D, Liu R, et al. Interactions between dyslipidemia and the immune system and their relevance as putative therapeutic targets in atherosclerosis. Pharmacology & Therapeutics. 2019;**193**:50-62

[184] Valanti EK, Dalakoura-Karagkouni K, Sanoudoi D. Current and emerging reconstituted HDL-apoA-I and HDL-apoE approaches to treat atherosclerosis. Journal of Personalized Medicine. 2018;**8**:34

[185] Wu D, Sharan C, Yang H, et al. Apolipoprotein E-deficient lipoproteins induce foam cell formation by downregulation of lysosomal hydrolases in macrophages. Journal of Lipid Research. 2007;**48**(12):2571-2578

[186] Stannard AK, Riddell DR, Sacre SM, et al. Cell-derived Apolipoprotein E (ApoE) particles inhibit vascular cell adhesion molecule-1 (VCAM-1) expression in human endothelial cells. The Journal of Biological Chemistry. 2001;**276**(49):46011-46016

[187] Mallat Z, Taleb S, Ait-Oufella H, Tedgui A. The role of adaptive T cell immunity in atherosclerosis. Journal of Lipid Research. 2009;**50**(Suppl):S364-S369

[188] Dose J, Huebble P, Nebel A, Rimbach G. APOE genotype and stress response—A mini review. Lipids in Health and Disease. 2016;**15**:121

[189] Zeleny M, Swertfeger DK, Weisgraber KH, Hui DY. Distinct apolipoprotein E isoform preference for inhibition of smooth muscle cell migration and proliferation. Biochemistry. 2002;**41**(39):11820-11823

[190] Yue L, Bian JT, Grizelj I, et al. ApoE enhances endothelial-NO production by modulating caveolin-1 interaction with eNOS. Hypertension. 2012;**60**(4):1040-1046

[191] Charo IS, Taub R. Anti-inflammatory therpeutics for the treatment of atherosclerosis. Nature Reviews. Drug Discovery. 2011;**10**(5):365-376

[192] Tardif JC, McMurray JJ, Klug E, et al. Effects of succinobucol (AGI-1067) after an acute coronary syndrome: A randomised, double-blind, placebo-controlled trial. Lancet. 2008;**371**(9626):1761-1768

[193] Rosenson RS. Phospholipase A2 inhibition and atherosclerotic vascular disease: Prospects for targeting secretory and lipoprotein-associated phospholipase A2 enzymes. Current Opinion in Lipidology. 2010;**21**(6):473-480

[194] Riccioni G, Zanasi A, Vitulano N, et al. Leukotrienes in atherosclerosis: New target inisights and future therapy perspectives. Mediators of Inflammation. 2009;**2009**:737282

[195] Lin J, Kakkar V, Lu X. Impact of MCP-1 in atherosclerosis. Current Pharmaceutical Design. 2014;**20**(28):4580-4588

[196] Tousoulis D, Oikonomou E, Economou EK, et al. Inflammatory cytokines in atherosclerosis: Current therapeutic approaches. European Heart Journal. 2016;**37**:1723-1735

Section 2

Dyslipidemia in Special Populations

Chapter 3

Dyslipidemia in Special Populations, the Elderly, Women, HIV, Chronic Kidney Disease and ESRD, and Minority Groups

Amarpali Brar, Jeans M. Santana, Moro O. Salifu and Clinton D. Brown

Abstract

This chapter discusses the management of dyslipidemia in special patient populations: the elderly, woman and pregnancy, renal disease, human immunodeficiency virus (HIV), and different racial/ethnic groups. In the elderly, dyslipidemia is often underdiagnosed and undertreated. Consideration for potential atherosclerotic risk-reduction benefits, risk of adverse effects, drug-drug interactions, and patient preferences should precede the initiation of statin therapy. Data on pregnant women are lacking and need future research. Dyslipidemia and its effects on the cardiovascular system in chronic kidney disease (CKD), end-stage renal disease (ESRD), and HIV are dynamic and multimodal. These conditions are states of chronic inflammation, where it is difficult to associate quantities of cholesterol types with outcomes. Among all racial groups, Asian Indians, Filipinos, and Hispanics are at a higher risk for dyslipidemia. Genetic differences in statin metabolism may explain this racial/ethnic difference.

Keywords: dyslipidemia, elderly, women, racial disparity, gender disparity

1. Introduction

Dyslipidemia, defined as high levels of low-density lipoprotein cholesterol (LDL-C) (≥130 mg/dl), total cholesterol (≥200 mg/dl), and triglycerides (TG) (≥150 mg/dl), or low levels of high-density lipoprotein cholesterol (HDL-C) [<40 (men) and < 50 (women) mg/dl], is a major risk factor for cardiovascular disease (CVD). Significant heterogeneity in patterns of dyslipidemia exists in these special populations. There is confusion among health-care providers regarding selection and implementation of appropriate guidelines, particularly for special patient populations. Patients in special populations may not clearly fall into one of the four statin-benefit groups identified by the ACC/AHA cholesterol guidelines [1].

In this chapter, we review the evidence in patterns of dyslipidemia and management in the elderly, women and pregnancy, CKD, ESRD, HIV, and different racial/ethnic groups.

IntechOpen

2. Dyslipidemia in the elderly

2.1 Epidemiology

According to census projections, the population age 65 and older is expected to double between 2012 and 2060, from 43.1 to 92.0 million [2]. CVD is the main cause of mortality in this age group. Lipid-lowering pharmacological intervention is one of the most successful cardiovascular preventative interventions. Concerns about its safety and efficacy in this age group have led different countries to adopt different strategies concerning the use of lipid-lowering drugs in the elderly [3]. In US population as reported in the National Health and Nutrition Examination Survey (NHANES) publications, across all age groups, triglyceride levels increase with age and reach a peak in men aged 50–59 years and in women aged 60–69 years. Apolipoprotein B (Apo B) and small dense LDLc also increase with age, while HDL-c does not seem to vary with age [4].

2.2 Management

Lifestyle modification including adhering to a heart healthy diet, regular exercise, avoidance of tobacco products, and maintenance of a healthy weight remains a critical component of ASCVD risk reduction.

2.2.1 Secondary prevention statin trials in elderly

In general, the elderly are usually underrepresented in published clinical trials. The only large randomized statin trials that focused on older patients are the Prospective Study of Pravastatin in the Elderly at Risk (PROSPER) and the Study Assessing Goals in the Elderly (SAGE) trial.

PROSPER is a randomized controlled trial in which 5804 patients aged 70–82 years with a history of, or risk factors for, vascular disease were randomized to receive pravastatin (40 mg/day; n = 2891) or placebo (n = 2913). Follow-up was 3.2 years. Pravastatin was found to reduce the incidence of coronary death, nonfatal myocardial infarction, and fatal or nonfatal stroke. Suggesting pravastatin may be utilized to manage dyslipidemia in the elderly and be prescribed to [5]. Later, the Study Assessing Goals in the Elderly (SAGE) compared the effect of intensive (atorvastatin 80 mg/day) with moderate (pravastatin 40 mg/day) cholesterol lowering with statins in a cohort of 893 patients, 65–85 years of age with coronary artery disease (CAD), and follow-up for 12 months. Atorvastatin-treated patients experienced greater LDL-C reductions than did pravastatin-treated patients, a trend toward fewer major acute cardiovascular events and a significantly greater reduction (77%) in all-cause death [6].

British Heart Foundation Heart Protection Study evaluated the role of simvastatin 40 mg/day versus placebo in 20,536 patients with coronary atherosclerosis and diabetics with coronary heart disease (CHD) risk equivalence. About 28% of randomized patients were ≥70 years of age. Among the 1263 individuals with 75–80 years of age at study entry, the rate of major coronary events in the simvastatin group was significantly lower than placebo group [7]. The long-term intervention with pravastatin in ischemic disease (LIPID) trial randomized patients with prior myocardial infarction or unstable angina to receive pravastatin 40 mg/day versus placebo, of which 39% (3514) were of age 65–75 years. Here, pravastatin reduced the risk for all CVD events, and similar adverse effects were observed in older and younger patients [8].

Other major secondary prevention trials, which included large numbers of elderly patients, are cholesterol and recurrent events (CARE) and Scandinavian simvastatin survival study (4S). In subgroup analyses of both studies, the absolute benefit of treatment was significantly greater in older patients as compared to younger patients for cardiovascular events [9, 10]. The 2013 ACC/AHA guidelines on the treatment of blood cholesterol to reduce atherosclerotic cardiovascular risk in adults recommended high-intensity statin therapy should be initiated or continued as first-line therapy in women and men ≤75 years of age who have clinical atherosclerotic cardiovascular disease (ASCVD), unless contraindicated. A larger amount of data supports the use of moderate-intensity statin therapy for secondary prevention in individuals with clinical ASCVD who are >75 years of age. However, the limited information available did not clearly support initiation of high-intensity statin therapy for secondary prevention in individuals >75 years of age [1]. Statin therapy to higher risk elderly patients is appropriate. In individuals with clinical ASCVD >75 years of age, practitioners should evaluate the potential for ASCVD risk-reduction benefits, adverse effects, drug-drug interactions and consider patient preferences when initiating a moderate- or high-intensity statin. It is reasonable to continue statin therapy in those who are tolerating it [1, 11]. Physicians treating the elderly must also consider the functional age of the patient and the impact of long-term drug therapy on safety and quality of life. Caution is recommended when statins are used in frail elderly patients, who may be more susceptible to drug-related myopathy and other side effects [12].

2.2.2 Primary prevention and statin trials

The Anglo-Scandinavian Cardiac Outcomes trial randomized 19,342 hypertensive patients (aged 40–79 years with at least three other cardiovascular risk factors) to be assigned to atorvastatin 10 mg or placebo. Nonfatal myocardial infarction and fatal cardiovascular disease were significantly lower in the statin group [13]. In a post hoc analysis, efficacy and safety of atorvastatin in 1129 patients aged 65–75 years at randomization was compared with 1709 younger patients in the Collaborative Atorvastatin Diabetes Study (CARDS). Primary end point of time to first occurrence of acute coronary heart disease events, coronary revascularizations, or stroke was similar in both groups. The overall safety profile of atorvastatin was similar between age groups [14]. Justification for the Use of statins in Prevention: An Intervention Trial Evaluating Rosuvastatin (JUPITER) is a randomized, double-blind, placebo-controlled trial with 17,802 participants of which 5695 were 70 years or older with LDL-C levels <130 mg/dl and high-sensitivity C-reactive protein levels of 2.0 mg/L or more without cardiovascular disease and were randomly assigned in a 1:1 ratio to receive 20 mg of rosuvastatin daily or placebo. In secondary analysis of this trial, no significant heterogeneity was found in treatment effects by age, absolute reductions in event rates associated with rosuvastatin were greater in elderly. The relative rate of any serious adverse event among older patients in the rosuvastatin versus placebo group was 1.05 (CI, 0.93–1.17) [15, 16].

As per 2013 ACC/AHA guideline on the treatment of blood cholesterol to reduce atherosclerotic cardiovascular risk in adults; four statin benefit groups are individuals with ASCVD, individuals with primary elevations of LDL-C ≥ 190 mg/day, individuals 40–75 years of age with diabetes and LDL-C 70 to 189 mg/dl without clinical ASCVD, and individuals without clinical ASCVD or diabetes who are 40–75 years of age and have LDL-C 70–189 mg/dl and an estimated 10-year ASCVD risk of ≥7.5%. This requires a clinician-patient discussion. Few data are available to indicate an ASCVD event reduction benefit in primary prevention among individuals >75 years of age who do not have clinical ASCVD. Therefore, initiation of statins for primary prevention of ASCVD in individuals >75 years of age requires consideration of additional factors, including increasing comorbidities, safety considerations, and priorities of care. The Pooled Cohort Equations can also provide information on expected 10-year ASCVD risk for those 76–79 years of age that may inform the treatment decision. A discussion of the potential ASCVD risk-reduction benefits, risk of adverse effects, drug-drug interactions, and consideration of patient preferences should precede the initiation of statin therapy for primary prevention in older individuals [1].

2.2.3 Statin and side effects

In the PROSPER study, no rhabdomyolysis or serum CK concentration > 10 times the upper limit of normal was reported. There was no statistically significant difference in the incidence of reported myalgia between the pravastatin and placebo groups (1.2 and 1.1%, respectively). In the SAGE study, incidence of myalgia was also not different between the atorvastatin and pravastatin treatment groups (3.1% versus 2.7%) with only one individual found to have CK level > 10 times the upper limit of normal in the pravastatin treatment group but none in the atorvastatin group [5, 6]. In a retrospective study, Graham et al. reported rhabdomyolysis risk was similar and low for monotherapy with atorvastatin, pravastatin, and simvastatin. Combined statin-fibrate use was associated with increased risk, especially in older patients with diabetes mellitus [17].

All of the available statins, with the exception of pravastatin and rosuvastatin, are metabolized by the cytochrome P450 (CYP) system. Serum concentrations of these statins can potentially be increased when other medications competing for the CYP system or CYP isoenzyme inhibitors are prescribed and can lead to increased risk of myositis and rhabdomyolysis. There is an age-related decrease in glomerular filtration rate, decrease in hepatic blood flow, decrease in drug clearance, and increased expression of P-glycoproteins resulting in alterations in the rate of drug transport across cellular membranes [18–20].

2.3 Other medications

2.3.1 Ezetimibe

Improved Reduction of Outcomes: Vytorin Efficacy International Trial (IMPROVE-IT) evaluated the effect of ezetimibe combined with simvastatin, as compared to simvastatin alone in 18,144 patients with acute coronary syndrome. Subgroup analysis showed a benefit of ezetimibe in the 7971 patients' over 65 years and 2798 patients' over 75 years of age [21].

2.3.2 Proprotein convertase subtilisin/kexin type 9 (PCSK9) inhibitors

The first large cardiovascular outcome study using PCSK9 inhibitor therapy (FOURIER) was a randomized, double-blind placebo-controlled trial of 27,564 subjects with 12,254 patients over the age 65 years with ASCVD and LDL-C levels ≥70 mg/dl while on maximally tolerated statin therapy, randomly assigned to receive evolocumab or placebo. In these patients, there was a significant decrease in composite outcome of cardiovascular death, myocardial infarction (MI), stroke, hospitalization for unstable angina, or coronary revascularization. However, cost is prohibitive for generalized use [22].

2.3.3. Fibrates

No data are available for fibrates in patients over 75 years of age. World Health Organization Clofibrate Study, Helsinki Heart Study (HHS), Bezafibrate Infarction Prevention (BIP), and Veterans Affairs Program High-Density Lipoprotein Cholesterol Intervention Trial (VA-HIT) showed reduction in the risk of myocardial infraction. Fenofibrate is considered the preferred agent, due to once-daily dosing and a favorable adverse reactions profile. Caution is needed in elderly patients with reduced renal function [23–26].

In conclusion, cardiovascular prevention clinical trial evidence for the patients over age 75 years is very limited. Management of dyslipidemia in the elderly requires consideration of comorbidities, safety considerations, polypharmacy, and priorities of care.

3. Dyslipidemia in women

3.1 Gender and cardiovascular risk

CVD is a major cause of death in women. While the risk of CVD in men increases after age 40 years, risk develops 7–10 years later in women. Incidence of CAD in premenopausal women is 3–4 times lower than in men [27, 28]. After menopause due to loss of vasodilating property of estrogen and increased sympathetic activity, the risk of CAD is increased and is similar to men [29–31]. Risk factors unique to women are use of oral contraceptives, menopause, hormone replacement therapy, gestational hypertension, and diabetes. Obesity and metabolic syndrome are also more prevalent in women [32].

Plasma cholesterol levels and LDL-C levels are similar in both sexes during the infancy and adolescence. LDL levels increase progressively in both men and women after the age of 20, but more rapidly in men. Size of the LDL particles reduces as men age, while it remains stable in women until menopause then becomes smaller [33].

3.2 Management of dyslipidemia

In 1999, American heart association (AHA) developed the first women-specific clinical report regarding recommendations for CVD prevention [34]. In the 2011 AHA update, effectiveness-based guidelines for the prevention of CVD in women recommended lifestyle approaches for LDL-C < 100 mg/dl, HDL-C > 50 mg/dl, triglycerides <150 mg/dl, and non-HDL-C (total cholesterol minus HDL) <130 mg/dl (class I recommendation; level of evidence B). LDL-C-lowering drug therapy with lifestyle therapy in women with coronary heart disease (CHD) to achieve an LDL-C < 100 mg/dl (class I; level of evidence A) and is also indicated in women with other atherosclerotic CHD or diabetes mellitus or 10-year absolute risk 20% (class I; level of evidence B). A reduction to <70 mg/dl is reasonable in very-high-risk women like those with recent acute coronary syndrome (ACS) or multiple cardiovascular risk factors with CHD and may require an LDL-lowering drug combination (class IIa; level of evidence B). In women >60 years of age and with an estimated CHD risk >10%, statins could be considered if hsCRP is >2 mg/dl after lifestyle modification and no acute inflammatory process is present (class IIb; level of evidence B). Niacin or fibrate therapy can be useful when HDL-C is low (<50 mg/dl) or non-HDL-C is elevated (>130 mg/dl) in high-risk women after LDL-C goal is reached (class IIb; level of evidence B) [35].

In 2013 ACC/AHA guidelines added, treatment decisions for women should be based on the level of ASCVD risk. Statin treatment based on estimated 10-year ASCVD risk avoids the overtreatment of lower risk groups, such as younger, non-Hispanic white women who, despite moderate elevations in LDL-C, are typically not at significantly increased risk for ASCVD in the absence of other substantial risk factors [1]. The European Atherosclerosis Society (ESC/EAS) recommends that assessment of CV risk should be gender specific and recommended statin therapy be initiated as primary and secondary prevention for women at high risk [36].

3.3 Women in hyperlipidemia clinical trials

Women have been underrepresented in many primary and secondary prevention trials. In major primary prevention trials, the number of women varied from 15 to 49%. In AFCAPS (15%), HPS (30%), ALLHAT-LLT (49%), and in ASCOT-LLA trial (19%) were women [37, 38]. In a prospective, randomized, open-labeled, blinded Japanese primary prevention trial of patients with hypercholesterolemia, 5547 (68%) were women randomly assigned to diet alone or diet with pravastatin daily. Treatment with a low dose of pravastatin reduced the risk of CHD but subgroup analysis of CHD risk in women was not statistically significant [39]. JUPITER trial participants included 6801 women ≥60 years of age and 11,001 men ≥50 years of age with high-sensitivity C-reactive protein ≥2 mg/L and LDL-C < 130 mg/dl, randomized to rosuvastatin versus placebo. JUPITER demonstrated that for primary prevention, rosuvastatin reduced CVD events in women with a relative risk reduction similar to that in men, a finding supported by meta-analysis of primary prevention statin trials [40].

In major secondary prevention trials, 4S included 827 (19% woman), CARE 576 (14%), LIPID 1516 (17%), TNT 1902 (19%), and SEARCH trial included 2052 (17%) women [41–44]. Cholesterol lowering with simvastatin produced similar reductions in relative risk for major coronary events in women compared with men. There were too few female deaths to assess the effects on mortality in women [41]. A meta-analysis of 13 large trials for a total of 11,435 women in primary prevention and 8272 in secondary prevention concluded that lipid lowering does not affect CHD mortality in women for primary prevention, but it is effective for secondary prevention [27].

3.4 Gender differences in statin use

Women are more likely to have poor lipid control. There have been conflicting results regarding gender differences in benefit of statins in women with CVD. However, in a meta-analysis performed on data from 22 trials of statin therapy versus control (n = 134,537) and five trials of more intensive versus less intensive statin therapy, 27% of 174,149 randomized participants were women. In men and women at an equivalent risk of cardiovascular disease, statin therapy was equally effective for the prevention of major vascular events. Kostis et al. performed a meta-analysis consisting of 18 randomized clinical trials of statins with gender-specific outcomes and found statin therapy was associated with significant decreases in cardiovascular events and in all-cause mortality in women and men [45].

There is a gender-specific impact of transporter polymorphisms on statin pharmacokinetics. Estrogen-induced water and sodium retention, increased volume for lipophilic drugs, higher protein-binding globulins, higher CYP3A4 activity, lower body mass index, and lower renal clearance in women may affect absorption of different statins. Women seem to be at greater risk of statin-induced rhabdomyolysis. In a US case-control study of 252,460 users of lipid-lowering therapy, there was trend for increased risk of rhabdomyolysis [46]. In the JUPITER study, the occurrence of serious adverse events was similar in both men and women [40].

3.5 Pregnancy

3.5.1 Normal changes in pregnancy

Metabolic adaptations during pregnancy are essential to meet the physiological demands of pregnancy as well as development of the fetus. An increase in insulin resistance results in increases in maternal glucose and free fatty acid concentrations, allowing for greater substrate availability for fetal growth. Production of progesterone leads to lipogenesis, lipids are transported across the placenta and metabolized; this signifies the essential role of lipids to normal fetal development [47, 48]. Within 6 weeks of gestation, lipid levels drop slightly followed by rise in both total cholesterol and marked increase in triglycerides (TG). HDL-C levels and apolipoprotein A-I levels also increase during normal gestation, with peak levels during the second trimester. As TG levels rise, there is a decrease in low-density lipoprotein (LDL) size with an increased proportion of atherogenic small-dense LDL. Both cholesterol and triglyceride concentrations decrease significantly within 24 h of delivery. However, while TG levels continued to decrease rapidly returning to nonpregnant levels during the puerperium, LDL-C remained elevated for at least 6–7 weeks postpartum [49, 50]. During pregnancy, lipoprotein Lp(a) levels increase with gestational age and fall to prepregnancy levels within 6 months postpartum [51, 52].

3.5.2 Lipids and complications in pregnancy

Preeclamptic women exhibit higher mean serum TG levels, elevated LDL-C fractions, increased levels of Lp(a), and lower HDL cholesterol levels compared with healthy pregnant women [49]. Amsterdam Born Children and Their Development (ABCD) cohort study showed that every unit increase in TG was linearly associated with an increased risk of preeclampsia, pregnancy-induced hypertension, and preterm delivery. Total cholesterol was not associated with any of the outcome measures [53]. Women who have higher concentrations of small-dense LDL fractions during pregnancy tend to have increased risk of cardiovascular disease later in life [53, 54].

In the multicenter, prospective Coronary Artery Risk Development in Young Adults study, 1010 women of which 49% identified as black with at least one singleton birth with 20 years of follow-up were evaluated. There was a U-shaped relationship between prepregnancy cholesterol concentrations and preterm birth risk with both low ((<156 mg/dl) and high cholesterol (>195 mg/dl) related to preterm birth risk [55]. Observational and experimental evidence increasingly supports a relation between growth and development during fetal and infant life and health in later years. Additionally, preterm newborns have been found to be at an increased risk of CVD later in life [56].

3.5.2.1 Antihyperlipidemia therapy

Pregnant women are generally excluded from clinic trials, thus the data are limited. HMG-CoA reductase inhibitors have been associated with teratogenicity and congenital malformation and are not recommended. Fibrates and nicotinic acid have not been well studied and are not recommended. Omega fatty acids, on the other hand, can be safely used as monotherapy to decrease TG levels.

4. Dyslipidemia in CKD and ESRD

4.1 Epidemiology and pathogenesis

Patients with CKD and ESRD are at an increased risk of CVD, and are more likely to die because of adverse cardiovascular events [57]. In addition to traditional risk factors like hypertension, diabetes mellitus, dyslipidemia, and a family history of CAD, patients with CKD are plagued by nontraditional risk factors like homocysteinemia, mineral bone disease, carbamylation, and chronic inflammation [58, 59]). As CKD progresses, an unstable vascular environment ensues which threatens endothelial function and lipoprotein integrity and thus potentiating adverse cardiovascular outcomes. **Figure 1** shows mechanism of dyslipidemia in this population.

Dyslipidemia in these patients is undoubtedly one of the strongest risk factors for these adverse cardiovascular outcomes. Despite these data, however, CVD remains underdiagnosed and undertreated in patients with CKD. Dyslipidemia has been found to be distinctly different from the general population and variable depending on the stage of CKD [60]. The lipid profile of patients with nondialysis-dependent CKD is usually composed of low HDL-C and high triglycerides with normal to low total cholesterol and low-density lipoprotein cholesterol [61]. In fact, plasma triglycerides start to increase in early stages of CKD and show the highest concentrations in nephrotic syndrome and in dialysis patients, especially those who are treated with peritoneal dialysis [60]. In patients with nondialysis-dependent CKD, the hypertriglyceridemia has been attributed to delayed catabolism and increased hepatic production of triglyceride-rich lipoproteins, and to a smaller extent by the presence of lipase inhibitors [62]. This altered catabolism in turn results in the accumulation of triglyceride-rich lipoproteins, like IDL and small-dense LDL (sdLDL) which are highly atherogenic [63, 64].

Though elevated LDL-C is not a typical feature of these patients, sdLDL, an LDL subtype, is increased and carries the ability to penetrate the vessel wall, becomes oxidized, and triggers the atherosclerotic process. The subfractions of HDL in CKD and ESRD are also different than that of the general population. In uremia [65], LDL and HDL, their subfractions, lipidomes, and proteomes, gradually become more susceptible to structural modifications such as carbamylation, oxidation, glycation, nitration, and homocysteinylation [66, 67]. Most of these effectors are irreversible and amplify the uptake by the scavenger receptors on the surface of macrophages [60]. HDL's vital components like ApoA-I, PON-1, and LCAT are altered, ultimately attenuating HDL's cyto- and vascular-protective properties [68] . The reduced

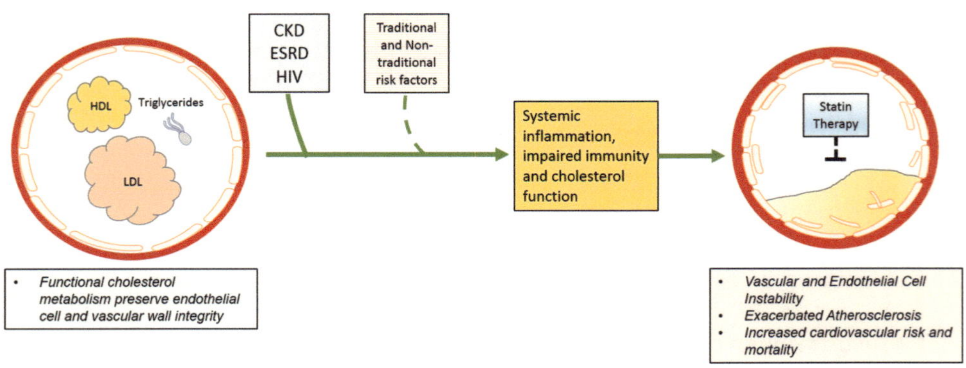

Figure 1.
Mechanism of dyslipidemia in chronic kidney disease (CKD), end stage renal disease (ESRD), and human immunodeficiency virus (HIV) patients.

PON-1 activity further predisposes LDL and HDL to more oxidation and, in turn, dysfunction and enhanced atherogenic potential [69]. In fact, it has been found that increasing serum HDL-C over time is paradoxically associated with significantly higher all-cause and cardiovascular mortality [70].

4.2 Management

Recent studies show that statin therapy can decrease cardiovascular mortality in CKD population. Heart Protection Study and Anglo-Scandinavian Cardiac Outcomes Trial (ASCOT) demonstrated that CKD patients treated with simvastatin exhibited a reduction of cardiovascular morbidity and mortality [71, 13]. Results from the Pravastatin Pooling Project showed similar cardioprotective effects [72]. Atorvastatin and rosuvastatin also reduced the relative risk of cardiovascular events in CKD patients and improved outcomes were found with higher atorvastatin doses [73–75]. Study of Heart and Renal Protection (SHARP) trial randomized 9270 patients with CKD with no prior history of CAD and found that simvastatin 20 mg plus ezetimibe 10 mg daily safely reduced the incidence of major atherosclerotic events in CKD patients [76].

KDIGO panel provides recommendations for dyslipidemia in patients at all stages of CKD based on a few large, randomized controlled trials and post hoc analyses of the subgroup of CKD patients from statin trials in the general population [76, 77]. In adult CKD patients ≥50 years age, statin therapy alone is recommended for those with GFR ≥ 60 ml/min and statin or statin/ezetimibe therapy is recommended for GFR < 60 ml/min. In adults aged 18–49 years with CKD, statin treatment is recommended in patients with known coronary disease, diabetes mellitus, prior ischemic stroke or estimated 10-year incidence of coronary death or nonfatal myocardial infarction >10%. Neither ACC/AHA nor KDIGO guidelines recommend initiation of statin therapy or combination treatment with statin and ezetimibe in dialysis-dependent patients on the basis of results from the AURORA (A Study to Evaluate the Use of Rosuvastatin in Subjects on Regular Hemodialysis: An Assessment of Survival and Cardiovascular Events) and Deutsche Diabetes Dialyse Studie (4-D) trials. However, patients already on lipid-lowering therapy at the time of progression to dialysis may continue treatment [76, 78–80].

Novel and innovative therapies are needed to address the multiple lipid/lipoprotein abnormalities that facilitate high cardiovascular risk and mortality in patients with dialysis-dependent CKD.

5. Dyslipidemia in renal transplant recipients

5.1 Epidemiology

Risk of cardiovascular events in kidney transplant recipients is markedly elevated as compared to people without CKD. Prevalence of hyperlipidemia ranges from 16 to 78% in kidney transplant recipients. Hypercholesterolemia has peak incidence at 12 months posttransplant and correlates with excessive body weight. After transplantation, increases in total cholesterol, LDL-C, very-low-density lipoprotein (VLDL)-cholesterol, and TG have been noted. In addition, LDL-C may be more susceptible to oxidation, making the particle more atherogenic. HDL-C levels may be normal or even high although the composition of HDL may not be normal [81].

5.2 Mechanisms of dyslipidemia

Immunosuppressive agents contribute significantly to hyperlipidemia in renal transplant recipients. Corticosteroids induce insulin resistance. Hyperinsulinemia leads to increased hepatic uptake of free fatty acids (FFA) which constitute the main substrate for VLDL cholesterol synthesis. There is increased conversion of VLDL to LDL cholesterol, leading to a rise in LDL cholesterol levels and downregulation of LDL receptors [81–83]. Calcineurin inhibitors interfere with binding of LDL-to-LDL receptor leading to increase in LDL-C, interfere with bile acid synthesis and lead to LDL receptor downregulation. Cyclosporine is highly lipophilic. Tacrolimus is associated with less hyperlipidemia [84]. Rapamycin inhibits lipoprotein lipase, associated with decrease in apolipoprotein-B 100 catabolism, and increases secretion of VLDL cholesterol [85]. Other secondary causes include nephrotic syndrome, hypothyroidism, diabetes mellitus, excessive alcohol intake, obesity, chronic liver disease, and genetic predisposition.

5.3 Management

Lipid profile evaluation including total cholesterol, LDL, HDL, and triglyceride levels is recommended. Kidney Disease Improving Global Outcomes (KDIGO) suggest treatment with statins in adult kidney transplant recipients [77]. Assessment of Lescol in Renal Transplantation (ALERT) trial is the only multicenter, randomized, double-blind, placebo-controlled trial in renal transplant recipients. In this study, 2102 renal transplant recipients with total cholesterol 4·0–9 mmol/l were randomized to receive fluvastatin (n = 1050) or placebo (n = 1052). After a mean follow-up of 5 years, fluvastatin lowered LDL cholesterol concentrations by 32%. Although cardiac deaths and nonfatal myocardial infarction seemed to be reduced, fluvastatin did not reduce rates of coronary intervention procedures or mortality [86]. Of 1787 patients who completed ALERT, 1652 (92%) were followed in the extension trial with mean follow-up of 6.7 years which showed 29% reduction in cardiac death or definite nonfatal myocardial infarction in the fluvastatin arm [87]. Due to the known interaction of calcineurin inhibitors through CYP3A isoenzyme system, lower doses of statins are generally used as compared to general population. Among fibrates, fenofibrate is less myotoxic than gemfibrozil when combined with statin but fenofibrate should be avoided in advanced CKD. Bile acid sequesterants are not widely used due to gastrointestinal side effects and can also interfere with absorption of immunosuppressants. Ezetimibe is considered safe in renal transplant recipients.

6. Dyslipidemia in HIV

Antiretroviral therapy (ART) has prolonged the survival of HIV-infected individuals, which, in effect, has increased the prevalence of comorbidities, like coronary heart disease. Studies have shown that HIV-infected individuals have higher cardiovascular disease (CVD) risk than uninfected persons in the United States [88–90]. Paisible et al. reported a 1.5–2-fold increased risk of incident myocardial infarction compared with uninfected subjects [91]. Among HIV patients, women have been found to have higher CVD risk than men [92]. Risk, however, cannot be attributed to HIV alone as traditional CVD risk factors like smoking [93], dyslipidemia, diabetes mellitus, and hypertension [92] have been found to be more common among those infected. **Table 1** summarizes the traditional and nontraditional risk factors for cardiovascular disease in special populations.

Their lipid profile is comprised of hypertriglyceridemia, increased sdLDL, and low HDL-C levels [94, 95]. Atheromas have been found to have larger lipid pools with dystrophic calcifications [96]. Consequently, the coronary arteries have a higher burden of coronary plaque and prevalence of detectable calcium [97–99]. These plaques are rupture-prone and associated with inflammation [100] and monocyte activation [101]. As a result, patients tend to have higher rates of subclinical vascular disease [102, 103]. ART-associated lipodystrophy has been linked with these cardiac and metabolic complications [104]. However, newer ART medications have had less effect on dyslipidemia and related myocardial events [105]. Still, CD4 cell depletion and immune dysfunction perpetuates HIV-related atherosclerosis, irrespective of ART [106]. Silverberg et al. reported that CD4 counts <200 cells/mm^3 were significantly associated with increased risk of MI [105]. While viral load and prior ART use were not associated with MI, unsuppressed HIV viremia was associated with MI [89] and stroke [107]. Dyslipidemia and its effects on the cardiovascular system in HIV are dynamic and multimodal. In these states of chronic inflammation, it is difficult to associate quantities of cholesterol types with outcomes. That is, in these special populations, there may not be a "good" or "bad" cholesterol, but rather dysfunctional lipoprotein atherosclerosis.

Studies have shown that statins are safe and beneficial in those infected with HIV; however, the use of statins remains relatively low [89, 108, 109]. Reasons include (1) the low prevalence of elevated LDL-C, (2) their uncertain efficacy for CVD prevention, and (3) the potential to adverse side effects and negative drug-drug interactions [80]. National Lipid Association (NLA) recommends that all HIV-infected patients be first assessed for cardiovascular risk and counseled about lifestyle interventions like diet, exercise, and smoking for the prevention of atherosclerotic cardiovascular disease. In addition, a fasting lipid panel should be obtained in all newly identified HIV-infected patients before and after starting antiretroviral therapy. TG >500 mg/dl that are refractory to lifestyle modification or changes in ART (if an option) should be treated with either a fibrate (fenofibrate preferred) or prescription omega-3 fatty acids to lower TG to <500 mg/dl. Non-HDL-C and

Traditional	Non-traditional		
	CKD	**HIV**	**Renal transplant**
Diabetes mellitus and insulin resistance	Hyperhomocysteinemia	Antiretroviral therapy	Immunosuppressive therapy: Glucocorticoids Calcineurin inhibitor Rapamycin
Hypertension	Hypercalcemia and hyperphosphatemia		
Dyslipidemia	Chronic inflammation and oxidative stress		
Obesity and physical inactivity	Anemia of chronic disease		
Smoking	Microalbuminuria		
Family history of atherosclerosis	Nephrotic syndrome		
Age			
Gender			

CKD, chronic kidney disease; HIV, human immunodeficiency virus.

Table 1.
Traditional and nontraditional risk factors for cardiovascular disease in special populations.

LDL-C should be reassessed for appropriate management with statin therapy with caution of drug-drug interactions and side effects. To this end, the NLA Expert Panel recommends clinicians to prescribe pitavastatin as the generally preferred agent in HIV-infected patients [80].

7. Racial differences in dyslipidemia

7.1 Epidemiology

National Health and Nutrition Examination Survey (NHANES) is the primary data source for national prevalence rates of dyslipidemia in the US with data on Whites, black/African Americans, and Hispanics/Latinos but is limited in data on Asian subgroups [110]. NHANES data in 2013 showed that the prevalence rate of high LDL-C was highest among Mexican men (40%) and women (30%), followed by non-Hispanic black men (33%) and women (31%). Non-Hispanic white men (30%) and women (29%) had the lowest prevalence of high LDL-C. The prevalence rates of low HDL were 20% in black men and 10% in black women as compared to prevalence rates among non-Hispanic white men (33%) and women (12%) and Hispanic American men (34%) and women (15%). NHANES data in 2008 reported prevalence of high TG in 35% of Hispanic Americans, 33% among non-Hispanic whites, and 16% among non-Hispanic blacks [111]. American Heart Association (AHA), in conjunction with the Centers for Disease Control and Prevention, and the National Institutes of Health reported prevalence of hyperlipidemia in non-Hispanic black men (32.6%) and non-Hispanic black women (36.1%), Hispanic men (43.1%), Hispanic women (41.2%), non-Hispanic white men (37%) and in women (43.4%) and for non-Hispanic Asians, prevalence was 39.9% in men and 40.5% in women [112]. Data from outpatient cohort of adults 35 years or older from 2008 to 2011 in northern California found that compared with non-Hispanic whites, every minority subgroup had an increased prevalence of high triglycerides except blacks. Most minority groups had an increased prevalence of low HDL-C, except for Japanese and blacks. The prevalence of HDL-C was increased among Asian Indians, Filipinos, Japanese, and Vietnamese compared with non-Hispanic whites [113]. **Table 2** shows cholesterol levels in minority populations compared to non-Hispanic Whites in the United States.

The Study of Health Assessment and Risk in Ethnic groups (SHARE), a prospective Canadian trial, showed that South Asians including Asian Indians had an increased prevalence of total cholesterol, high LDL-C, low HDL-C, and high TG compared to European and Chinese cohort [114]. The Multi-Ethnic Study of Atherosclerosis (MESA), a multicenter cohort study of 6814 adults aged 45 to 84 years who were free of clinical CVD at baseline were evaluated for CVD risk and self-reported use of lipid-lowering therapy. Black and Hispanic Americans had prevalence of dyslipidemia that was comparable to that of non-Hispanic whites but were less likely to be treated and controlled. Ethnic disparities were attenuated substantially by adjustment for health-care access variables [115]. Data from the Hispanic Community Health Study (HCHS)/Study of Latinos (SOL), an observational study, showed high prevalence of dyslipidemia among Central American men and Puerto Rican women [116].

7.2 Dyslipidemia and cardiovascular outcomes

In the US, cardiovascular mortality rates are highest in blacks as compared to Hispanics [117]. An early study of CHD among Japanese migrants compared with

	Percent of population	Total cholesterol	HDL	LDL	TGs	Lp(a)	ASCVD
Hispanics							
Men	17%	↑	↓	↑	↑	↔	↑
Women		↓					
African Americans							
Men	13%	↔	↑	↓	↓	↑	↑
Women		↔		↔			
Asians *(data limited)*	6%	↑	↓	↑	↑	–	↑
American Indians/ Alaska Natives *(data limited)*	2%	–	↑	–	–	–	↑

HDL, high-density lipoprotein; LDL, low-density lipoprotein; Lp(a), lipoprotein (a), ASCVD, atherosclerotic cardiovascular disease.

Table 2.
Cholesterol levels in minority populations compared to non-Hispanic Whites in the United States.

Japanese living in Japan showed higher rates of CAD in Japanese immigrants in America [118]. In a study of immigrant Asian Indian men in US, Enas et al. reported high prevalence of CAD, low HDL-C levels, and hypertriglyceridemia. Authors suggested "insulin resistance" as a common pathogenetic mechanism [119]. Increased risk of CAD in south Asian community was seen in data from other studies as well [114, 120, 121].

The 2013 ACC-AHA guidelines for the treatment of cholesterol expand the indications for statin therapy for the prevention of CVD. Ten-year ASCVD risk assessment calculator has been added to determine statin use [122]. ASCVD risk calculator is derived from cohorts that included African-American or white participants with at least 12 years of follow-up. Data from other racial/ethnic groups were insufficient, precluding their inclusion in the final analyses. The equations were also assessed in external validation studies with data from other available cohorts [123]. For other ethnic groups, ACC/AHA recommends use of the equations for non-Hispanic whites, though it acknowledges that estimates may underestimate the risk for American Indians, some Asian Americans (e.g., of south Asian ancestry), and some Hispanics (e.g., Puerto Ricans), and may overestimate the risk for others, including some Asian Americans (e.g., of east Asian ancestry) and some Hispanics (e.g., Mexican Americans) [124].

7.3 Statin metabolism

There are several genetic variants associated with altered statin metabolism. Single-nucleotide polymorphisms in the genes that encode the organic anion-transporting polypeptide (OATP) 1B1 (521 T > C), which regulates hepatic uptake of statins, and the adenosine triphosphate-binding cassette G2 (ABCG2) transporter (421C > A), which regulates hepatic efflux, have been reported [125–127]. Plasma exposure to rosuvastatin and its metabolites was significantly higher in Chinese, Malay, and Asian-Indian subjects compared with white subjects living in Singapore [128]. Rosuvastatin, a HMG-CoA reductase inhibitor, is excreted into bile mediated by breast cancer resistance protein (BCRP). BCRP 421C > A polymorphism may play an important role in the pharmacokinetics of rosuvastatin in healthy Chinese males [129]. In a Japanese study, single-nucleotide polymorphisms in OATP-C, such as T521C (Val174Ala), has been reported to be associated with altered pharmacokinetics of pravastatin [125]. In a US-based study cohort of 69 European-Americans and 38 African-Americans, SLCO1B1 genotype, in particular, the 521C allele, had a significant effect on the pharmacokinetics of pravastatin. European-Americans demonstrated significantly higher pravastatin levels as compared to African-Americans [130]. There is less information on statin metabolism in other racial/ethnic minority groups. In a randomized placebo-controlled trial of 25,673 patients, the absolute risk of myopathy with adding niacin-laropiprant to statin-based LDL cholesterol-lowering therapy was more than 10 times as great among Chinese as compared to their European counterparts [131]. The relative risk of myopathy with niacin-laropiprant versus placebo was also higher in Chinese patients [132].

Lifestyle risk factors include unhealthy diet, obesity, and physical inactivity. Racial/ethnic disparities also exist in these lifestyle risk factors. According to the National Health Interview Survey (NHIS) 2008–2010, Asian adults were less likely to be current smokers or to be obese. Black adults were more likely to be physically inactive, to be obese, and to get insufficient sleep. Hispanics were less likely than non-Hispanic adults to smoke cigarettes, get insufficient sleep, but were more likely to be inactive in terms of aerobic and muscle-strengthening leisure time. Immigration and acculturation have a profound impact on lifestyle in both Hispanics and Asians in the US [133]. Asian Indian, Filipino, Vietnamese women, and Asian Indian men have increased risk dyslipidemias as compared to non-Hispanic whites. Further research is needed to determine the role of dyslipidemia subtypes and other risk factors in explaining the higher risk of CVD in minority subgroups. By understanding these differences, clinicians will be able to provide more culturally competent recommendations on prevention and management of dyslipidemia.

8. Conclusion

In conclusion, differences in dyslipidemia patterns, risk factors, and management exist in the elderly, women and pregnancy, CKD, ESRD, HIV, and different racial ethnic groups. Nevertheless, they are frequently underrepresented in clinical trials, which calls for more inclusive research that will develop stronger recommendations of daily practice.

Author details

Amarpali Brar*, Jeans M. Santana, Moro O. Salifu and Clinton D. Brown
SUNY Downstate Medical Center, Brooklyn, NY, USA

*Address all correspondence to: amarpali.brar@downstate.edu

References

[1] Stone NJ, Robinson JG, Lichtenstein AH, Bairey Merz CN, Blum CB, Eckel RH, et al. 2013 ACC/AHA guideline on the treatment of blood cholesterol to reduce atherosclerotic cardiovascular risk in adults: A report of the American College of Cardiology/American Heart Association Task Force on Practice Guidelines. Circulation. 2014;**129** (25 Suppl 2):S1-S45 (Epub Nov 14, 2013)

[2] Sandra LC, Ortman JM. Projections of the size and composition of the U.S. population: 2014 to 2060. Current Population Reports. Washington, DC: U.S. Census Bureau; 2014:25-1143

[3] Streja D, Streja E. Management of dyslipidemia in the elderly. In: De Groot LJ, Chrousos G, Dungan K, Feingold KR, Grossman A, Hershman JM, et al., editors. Endotext. South Dartmouth (MA): MDText.com, Inc.; 2000

[4] Ghandehari H, Kamal-Bahl S, Wong ND. Prevalence and extent of dyslipidemia and recommended lipid levels in US adults with and without cardiovascular comorbidities: The National Health and Nutrition Examination Survey 2003-2004. American Heart Journal. 2008;**156**(1):112-119 (Epub Jul 1, 2008)

[5] Shepherd J, Blauw GJ, Murphy MB, Bollen EL, Buckley BM, Cobbe SM, et al. Pravastatin in elderly individuals at risk of vascular disease (PROSPER): A randomised controlled trial. Lancet. 2002;**360**(9346):1623-1630 (Epub Nov 30, 2002)

[6] Deedwania P, Stone PH, Bairey Merz CN, Cosin-Aguilar J, Koylan N, Luo D, et al. Effects of intensive versus moderate lipid-lowering therapy on myocardial ischemia in older patients with coronary heart disease: Results of the Study Assessing Goals in the Elderly (SAGE). Circulation. 2007;**115**(6): 700-707 (Epub Feb 7, 2007)

[7] Collins R, Armitage J, Parish S, Sleigh P, Peto R. MRC/BHF Heart Protection Study of cholesterol-lowering with simvastatin in 5963 people with diabetes: A randomised placebo-controlled trial. Lancet. 2003;**361**(9374):2005-2016 (Epub Jun 20, 2003)

[8] Prevention of cardiovascular events and death with pravastatin in patients with coronary heart disease and a broad range of initial cholesterol levels. The New England Journal of Medicine. 1998;**339**(19):1349-1357 (Epub Dec 5, 1998)

[9] Sacks FM, Pfeffer MA, Moye LA, Rouleau JL, Rutherford JD, Cole TG, et al. The effect of pravastatin on coronary events after myocardial infarction in patients with average cholesterol levels. Cholesterol and recurrent events trial investigators. The New England Journal of Medicine. 1996;**335**(14):1001-1009 (Epub Oct 3, 1996)

[10] Pedersen T et al. Randomised trial of cholesterol lowering in 4444 patients with coronary heart disease: The Scandinavian Simvastatin Survival Study (4S). Lancet. 1994;**344**(8934):1383-1389 (Epub Nov 19, 1994)

[11] Jacobson TA. Overcoming 'ageism' bias in the treatment of hypercholesterolaemia : A review of safety issues with statins in the elderly. Drug Safety. 2006;**29**(5):421-448 (Epub May 13, 2006)

[12] Pasternak RC, Smith SC Jr, Bairey-Merz CN, Grundy SM, Cleeman JI, Lenfant C. ACC/AHA/NHLBI clinical advisory on the use and safety of statins. Circulation. 2002;**106**(8):1024-1028 (Epub Aug 21, 2002)

[13] Sever PS, Dahlof B, Poulter NR, Wedel H, Beevers G, Caulfield M, et al.

Prevention of coronary and stroke events with atorvastatin in hypertensive patients who have average or lower-than-average cholesterol concentrations, in the Anglo-Scandinavian Cardiac Outcomes Trial—Lipid Lowering Arm (ASCOT-LLA): A multicentre randomised controlled trial. Lancet. 2003;**361**(9364):1149-1158 (Epub Apr 11, 2003)

[14] Neil HA, DeMicco DA, Luo D, Betteridge DJ, Colhoun HM, Durrington PN, et al. Analysis of efficacy and safety in patients aged 65-75 years at randomization: Collaborative Atorvastatin Diabetes Study (CARDS). Diabetes Care. 2006;**29**(11):2378-2384 (Epub Oct 27, 2006)

[15] Ridker PM, Danielson E, Fonseca FA, Genest J, Gotto AM Jr, Kastelein JJ, et al. Rosuvastatin to prevent vascular events in men and women with elevated C-reactive protein. The New England Journal of Medicine. 2008;**359**(21):2195-2207 (Epub Nov 11, 2008)

[16] Glynn RJ, Koenig W, Nordestgaard BG, Shepherd J, Ridker PM. Rosuvastatin for primary prevention in older persons with elevated C-reactive protein and low to average low-density lipoprotein cholesterol levels: Exploratory analysis of a randomized trial. Annals of Internal Medicine. 2010;**152**(8):488-496, W174 (Epub Apr 21, 2010)

[17] Graham DJ, Staffa JA, Shatin D, Andrade SE, Schech SD, La Grenade L, et al. Incidence of hospitalized rhabdomyolysis in patients treated with lipid-lowering drugs. The Journal of the American Medical Association. 2004;**292**(21):2585-2590 (Epub Dec 2, 2004)

[18] Cockcroft DW, Gault MH. Prediction of creatinine clearance from serum creatinine. Nephron. 1976;**16**(1):31-41 (Epub Jan 1, 1976)

[19] Wynne HA, Cope LH, Mutch E, Rawlins MD, Woodhouse KW, James OF. The effect of age upon liver volume and apparent liver blood flow in healthy man. Hepatology. 1989;**9**(2):297-301 (Epub Feb 1, 1989)

[20] Gupta S. P-glycoprotein expression and regulation. Age-related changes and potential effects on drug therapy. Drugs & Aging. 1995;**7**(1):19-29 (Epub Jul 1, 1995)

[21] Cannon CP, Blazing MA, Giugliano RP, McCagg A, White JA, Theroux P, et al. Ezetimibe added to statin therapy after acute coronary syndromes. The New England Journal of Medicine. 2015;**372**(25):2387-2397 (Epub Jun 4, 2015)

[22] Sabatine MS, Giugliano RP, Keech AC, Honarpour N, Wiviott SD, Murphy SA, et al. Evolocumab and clinical outcomes in patients with cardiovascular disease. The New England Journal of Medicine. 2017;**376**(18):1713-1722 (Epub Mar 18, 2017)

[23] Neve BP, Fruchart JC, Staels B. Role of the peroxisome proliferator-activated receptors (PPAR) in atherosclerosis. Biochemical Pharmacology. 2000;**60**(8):1245-1250 (Epub Sep 29, 2000)

[24] Rubins HB, Robins SJ, Collins D, Fye CL, Anderson JW, Elam MB, et al. Gemfibrozil for the secondary prevention of coronary heart disease in men with low levels of high-density lipoprotein cholesterol. Veterans affairs high-density lipoprotein cholesterol intervention trial study group. The New England Journal of Medicine. 1999;**341**(6):410-418 (Epub Aug 7, 1999)

[25] Frick MH, Elo O, Haapa K, Heinonen OP, Heinsalmi P, Helo P, et al. Helsinki Heart Study: Primary-prevention trial with gemfibrozil in

middle-aged men with dyslipidemia. Safety of treatment, changes in risk factors, and incidence of coronary heart disease. The New England Journal of Medicine. 1987;**317**(20):1237-1245 (Epub Nov 12, 1987)

[26] Brunner D, Agmon J, Kaplinsky E, et al. Secondary prevention by raising HDL cholesterol and reducing triglycerides in patients with coronary artery disease. Circulation. 2000;**102**(1):21-27 (Epub Jul 6, 2000)

[27] Walsh JM, Pignone M. Drug treatment of hyperlipidemia in women. The Journal of the American Medical Association. 2004;**291**(18):2243-2252 (Epub May 13, 2004)

[28] Mosca L, Banka CL, Benjamin EJ, Berra K, Bushnell C, Dolor RJ, et al. Evidence-based guidelines for cardiovascular disease prevention in women: 2007 update. Circulation. 2007;**115**(11):1481-1501 (Epub Feb 21, 2007)

[29] Wenger NK. Coronary disease in women. Annual Review of Medicine. 1985;**36**:285-294 (Epub Jan 1, 1985)

[30] Mucha L, Stephenson J, Morandi N, Dirani R. Meta-analysis of disease risk associated with smoking, by gender and intensity of smoking. Gender Medicine. 2006;**3**(4):279-291 (Epub Jun 22, 2007)

[31] Mercuro G, Longu G, Zoncu S, Cherchi A. Impaired forearm blood flow and vasodilator reserve in healthy postmenopausal women. American Heart Journal. 1999;**137**(4 Pt 1):692-697 (Epub Mar 31, 1999)

[32] Pavanello C, Mombelli G. Considering gender in prescribing statins: What do physicians need to know? Clinical Lipidology. 2015;**10**(6):499-512

[33] Kreisberg RA, Kasim S. Cholesterol metabolism and aging. The American Journal of Medicine. 1987;**82**(1B):54-60 (Epub Jan 26, 1987)

[34] Mosca L, Grundy SM, Judelson D, King K, Limacher M, Oparil S, et al. Guide to preventive cardiology for women. AHA/ACC scientific statement consensus panel statement. Circulation. 1999;**99**(18):2480-2484 (Epub May 11, 1999)

[35] Mosca L, Benjamin EJ, Berra K, Bezanson JL, Dolor RJ, Lloyd-Jones DM, et al. Effectiveness-based guidelines for the prevention of cardiovascular disease in women—2011 update: A guideline from the american heart association. Circulation. 2011;**123**(11):1243-1262 (Epub Feb 18, 2011)

[36] Reiner Z, Catapano AL, De Backer G, Graham I, Taskinen MR, Wiklund O, et al. ESC/EAS guidelines for the management of dyslipidaemias: The task force for the management of dyslipidaemias of the European Society of Cardiology (ESC) and the European Atherosclerosis Society (EAS). European Heart Journal. 2011;**32**(14):1769-1818 (Epub Jun 30, 2011)

[37] Downs JR, Clearfield M, Weis S, Whitney E, Shapiro DR, Beere PA, et al. Primary prevention of acute coronary events with lovastatin in men and women with average cholesterol levels: Results of AFCAPS/TexCAPS. Air Force/Texas Coronary Atherosclerosis Prevention Study. The journal of the American Medical Association. 1998;**279**(20):1615-1622 (Epub Jun 5, 1998)

[38] ALLHAT Collaborative Research Group authors. Major outcomes in moderately hypercholesterolemic, hypertensive patients randomized to pravastatin vs. usual care: The Antihypertensive and Lipid-Lowering Treatment to Prevent Heart Attack Trial (ALLHAT-LLT). The journal of the American Medical Association. 2002;**288**(23):2998-3007. (Epub Dec 20, 2002)

[39] Nakamura H, Arakawa K, Itakura H, Kitabatake A, Goto Y, Toyota T, et al. Primary prevention of cardiovascular disease with pravastatin in Japan (MEGA Study): A prospective randomised controlled trial. Lancet. 2006;**368**(9542):1155-1163 (Epub Oct 3, 2006)

[40] Mora S, Glynn RJ, Hsia J, MacFadyen JG, Genest J, Ridker PM. Statins for the primary prevention of cardiovascular events in women with elevated high-sensitivity C-reactive protein or dyslipidemia: Results from the Justification for the Use of Statins in Prevention: An Intervention Trial Evaluating Rosuvastatin (JUPITER) and meta-analysis of women from primary prevention trials. Circulation. 2010;**121**(9):1069-1077 (Epub Feb 24, 2010)

[41] Miettinen TA, Pyorala K, Olsson AG, Musliner TA, Cook TJ, Faergeman O, et al. Cholesterol-lowering therapy in women and elderly patients with myocardial infarction or angina pectoris: Findings from the Scandinavian Simvastatin Survival Study (4S). Circulation. 1997;**96**(12):4211-4218 (Epub Jan 7, 1998)

[42] Plehn JF, Davis BR, Sacks FM, Rouleau JL, Pfeffer MA, Bernstein V, et al. Reduction of stroke incidence after myocardial infarction with pravastatin: The Cholesterol and Recurrent Events (CARE) study. The care investigators. Circulation. 1999;**99**(2):216-223 (Epub Jan 20, 1999)

[43] Hague W, Forder P, Simes J, Hunt D, Tonkin A. Effect of pravastatin on cardiovascular events and mortality in 1516 women with coronary heart disease: Results from the Long-Term Intervention with Pravastatin in Ischemic Disease (LIPID) study. American Heart Journal. 2003;**145**(4):643-651 (Epub Apr 8, 2003)

[44] Link E, Parish S, Armitage J, Bowman L, Heath S, Matsuda F, et al. SLCO1B1 variants and statin-induced myopathy—A genomewide study. The New England Journal of Medicine. 2008;**359**(8):789-799 (Epub Jul 25, 2008)

[45] Kostis WJ, Cheng JQ, Dobrzynski JM, Cabrera J, Kostis JB. Meta-analysis of statin effects in women versus men. Journal of the American College of Cardiology. 2012;**59**(6):572-582 (Epub Feb 24, 2012)

[46] Schech S, Graham D, Staffa J, Andrade SE, La Grenade L, Burgess M, et al. Risk factors for statin-associated rhabdomyolysis. Pharmacoepidemiology and Drug Safety. 2007;**16**(3):352-358 (Epub Aug 8, 2006)

[47] Hadden DR, McLaughlin C. Normal and abnormal maternal metabolism during pregnancy. Seminars in Fetal & Neonatal Medicine. 2009;**14**(2):66-71 (Epub Nov 7, 2008)

[48] Lain KY, Catalano PM. Metabolic changes in pregnancy. Clinical Obstetrics and Gynecology. 2007;**50**(4):938-948 (Epub Nov 6, 2007)

[49] Belo L, Caslake M, Gaffney D, Santos-Silva A, Pereira-Leite L, Quintanilha A, et al. Changes in LDL size and HDL concentration in normal and preeclamptic pregnancies. Atherosclerosis. 2002;**162**(2):425-432 (Epub May 9, 2002)

[50] Potter JM, Nestel PJ. The hyperlipidemia of pregnancy in normal and complicated pregnancies. American Journal of Obstetrics and Gynecology. 1979;**133**(2):165-170 (Epub Jan 15, 1979)

[51] Fanshawe AE, Ibrahim M. The current status of lipoprotein (a) in pregnancy: A literature review. Journal of Cardiology. 2013;**61**(2):99-106 (Epub Nov 21, 2012)

[52] Manten GT, Franx A, van der Hoek YY, Hameeteman TM, Voorbij HA, Smolders HC, et al. Changes of plasma

lipoprotein(a) during and after normal pregnancy in Caucasians. The Journal of Maternal-Fetal & Neonatal Medicine : The Official Journal of the European Association of Perinatal Medicine, the Federation of Asia and Oceania Perinatal Societies, the International Society of Perinatal Obstet. 2003;**14**(2):91-95 (Epub Nov 25, 2003)

[53] Vrijkotte TG, Krukziener N, Hutten BA, Vollebregt KC, van Eijsden M, Twickler MB. Maternal lipid profile during early pregnancy and pregnancy complications and outcomes: The ABCD study. The Journal of Clinical Endocrinology and Metabolism. 2012;**97**(11):3917-3925 (Epub Aug 31, 2012)

[54] Enquobahrie DA, Williams MA, Butler CL, Frederick IO, Miller RS, Luthy DA. Maternal plasma lipid concentrations in early pregnancy and risk of preeclampsia. American Journal of Hypertension. 2004;**17**(7):574-581 (Epub Jul 6, 2004)

[55] Catov JM, Ness RB, Wellons MF, Jacobs DR, Roberts JM, Gunderson EP. Prepregnancy lipids related to preterm birth risk: The coronary artery risk development in young adults study. The Journal of Clinical Endocrinology and Metabolism. 2010;**95**(8):3711-3718 (Epub May 27, 2010)

[56] Gluckman PD, Hanson MA, Cooper C, Thornburg KL. Effect of in utero and early-life conditions on adult health and disease. The New England Journal of Medicine. 2008;**359**(1):61-73 (Epub Jul 4, 2008)

[57] Hemmelgarn BR, Clement F, Manns BJ, Klarenbach S, James MT, Ravani P, et al. Overview of the Alberta kidney disease network. BMC Nephrology. 2009;**10**:30 (Epub Oct 21, 2009)

[58] Ahmed MH, Khalil AA. Ezetimibe as a potential treatment for dyslipidemia associated with chronic renal failure and renal transplant. Saudi Journal of Kidney Diseases and Transplantation: An Official Publication of the Saudi Center for Organ Transplantation, Saudi Arabia. 2010;**21**(6):1021-1029 (Epub Nov 10, 2010)

[59] Holzer M, Zangger K, El-Gamal D, Binder V, Curcic S, Konya V, et al. Myeloperoxidase-derived chlorinating species induce protein carbamylation through decomposition of thiocyanate and urea: Novel pathways generating dysfunctional high-density lipoprotein. Antioxidants & Redox Signaling. 2012;**17**(8):1043-1052 (Epub Apr 3, 2012)

[60] Kwan BC, Kronenberg F, Beddhu S, Cheung AK. Lipoprotein metabolism and lipid management in chronic kidney disease. Journal of the American Society of Nephrology. 2007;**18**(4):1246-1261 (Epub Mar 16, 2007)

[61] Mikolasevic I, Zutelija M, Mavrinac V, Orlic L. Dyslipidemia in patients with chronic kidney disease: Etiology and management. International Journal of Nephrology and Renovascular Disease. 2017;**10**:35-45 (Epub Feb 23, 2017)

[62] Batista MC, Welty FK, Diffenderfer MR, Sarnak MJ, Schaefer EJ, Lamon-Fava S, et al. Apolipoprotein A-I, B-100, and B-48 metabolism in subjects with chronic kidney disease, obesity, and the metabolic syndrome. Metabolism: Clinical and Experimental. 2004;**53**(10):1255-1261 (Epub Sep 18, 2004)

[63] McNamara JR, Shah PK, Nakajima K, Cupples LA, Wilson PW, Ordovas JM, et al. Remnant-like particle (RLP) cholesterol is an independent cardiovascular disease risk factor in women: Results from the Framingham heart study. Atherosclerosis. 2001;**154**(1):229-236 (Epub Jan 4, 2001)

[64] Oi K, Hirano T, Sakai S, Kawaguchi Y, Hosoya T. Role of hepatic lipase in

intermediate-density lipoprotein and small, dense low-density lipoprotein formation in hemodialysis patients. Kidney International Supplement. 1999;**71**:S227-S228 (Epub Jul 21, 1999)

[65] Koch M, Kutkuhn B, Trenkwalder E, Bach D, Grabensee B, Dieplinger H, et al. Apolipoprotein B, fibrinogen, HDL cholesterol, and apolipoprotein(a) phenotypes predict coronary artery disease in hemodialysis patients. Journal of the American Society of Nephrology. 1997;**8**(12):1889-1898 (Epub Dec 24, 1997)

[66] Ikewaki K, Schaefer JR, Frischmann ME, Okubo K, Hosoya T, Mochizuki S, et al. Delayed in vivo catabolism of intermediate-density lipoprotein and low-density lipoprotein in hemodialysis patients as potential cause of premature atherosclerosis. Arteriosclerosis, Thrombosis, and Vascular Biology. 2005;**25**(12):2615-2622 (Epub Oct 1, 2005)

[67] Miljkovic M, Stefanovic A, Simic-Ogrizovic S, Vekic J, Bogavac-Stanojevic N, Cerne D, et al. Association of dyslipidemia, oxidative stress, and inflammation with redox status in VLDL, LDL, and HDL lipoproteins in patients with renal disease. Angiology. 2018;**69**(10):861-870. (Epub Jun 19, 2018)

[68] Santana JM, Brown CD. High-density lipoprotein carbamylation and dysfunction in vascular disease. Frontiers in Bioscience (Landmark Ed). 2018;**23**:2227-2234 (Epub May 18, 2018)

[69] Dantoine TF, Debord J, Charmes JP, Merle L, Marquet P, Lachatre G, et al. Decrease of serum paraoxonase activity in chronic renal failure. Journal of the American Society of Nephrology. 1998;**9**(11):2082-2088 (Epub Nov 10, 1998)

[70] Chang TI, Streja E, Soohoo M, Ko GJ, Rhee CM, Kovesdy CP, et al. Increments in serum high-density lipoprotein cholesterol over time are not associated with improved outcomes in incident hemodialysis patients. Journal of Clinical Lipidology. 2018;**12**(2):488-497 (Epub Feb 20, 2018)

[71] Heart Protection Study Collaborative Group authors. MRC/BHF Heart Protection Study of cholesterol lowering with simvastatin in 20,536 high-risk individuals: A randomised placebo-controlled trial. Lancet. 2002;**360**(9326): 7-22. (Epub Jul 13, 2002)

[72] Tonelli M, Isles C, Curhan GC, Tonkin A, Pfeffer MA, Shepherd J, et al. Effect of pravastatin on cardiovascular events in people with chronic kidney disease. Circulation. 2004;**110**(12): 1557-1563 (Epub Sep 15, 2004)

[73] Koren MJ, Davidson MH, Wilson DJ, Fayyad RS, Zuckerman A, Reed DP. Focused atorvastatin therapy in managed-care patients with coronary heart disease and CKD. American Journal of Kidney Diseases :The Official Journal of the National Kidney Foundation. 2009;**53**(5):741-750 (Epub Feb 14, 2009)

[74] Shepherd J, Kastelein JJ, Bittner V, Deedwania P, Breazna A, Dobson S, et al. Effect of intensive lipid lowering with atorvastatin on renal function in patients with coronary heart disease: The treating to new targets (TNT) study. Clinical Journal of the American Society of Nephrology. 2007;**2**(6): 1131-1139 (Epub Oct 19, 2007)

[75] Ridker PM, Macfadyen JG, Nordestgaard BG, Koenig W, Kastelein JJ, Genest J, et al. Rosuvastatin for primary prevention among individuals with elevated high-sensitivity c-reactive protein and 5% to 10% and 10% to 20% 10-year risk. Implications of the Justification for Use of Statins in Prevention: An Intervention Trial Evaluating Rosuvastatin (JUPITER)

trial for "intermediate risk". Circulation Cardiovascular Quality and Outcomes. 2010;**3**(5):447-452 (Epub Aug 26, 2010)

[76] Baigent C, Landray MJ, Reith C, Emberson J, Wheeler DC, Tomson C, et al. The effects of lowering LDL cholesterol with simvastatin plus ezetimibe in patients with chronic kidney disease (Study of Heart and Renal Protection): A randomised placebo-controlled trial. Lancet. 2011;**377**(9784):2181-2192 (Epub Jun 15, 2011)

[77] Tonelli M, Wanner C. Lipid management in chronic kidney disease: Synopsis of the kidney disease: Improving global outcomes 2013 clinical practice guideline. Annals of Internal Medicine. 2014;**160**(3):182 (Epub Dec 11, 2013)

[78] Fellstrom BC, Jardine AG, Schmieder RE, Holdaas H, Bannister K, Beutler J, et al. Rosuvastatin and cardiovascular events in patients undergoing hemodialysis. The New England Journal of Medicine. 2009;**360**(14):1395-1407 (Epub Apr 1, 2009)

[79] Wanner C, Krane V, Marz W, Olschewski M, Asmus HG, Kramer W, et al. Randomized controlled trial on the efficacy and safety of atorvastatin in patients with type 2 diabetes on hemodialysis (4D study): Demographic and baseline characteristics. Kidney & Blood Pressure Research. 2004;**27**(4):259-266 (Epub Aug 19, 2004)

[80] Jacobson TA, Maki KC, Orringer CE, Jones PH, Kris-Etherton P, Sikand G, et al. National lipid association recommendations for patient-centered management of dyslipidemia: Part 2. Journal of Clinical Lipidology. 2015;**9**(6 Suppl):S1-122.e1 (Epub Dec 25, 2015)

[81] Kobashigawa JA, Kasiske BL. Hyperlipidemia in solid organ transplantation. Transplantation. 1997;**63**(3):331-338 (Epub Feb 15, 1997)

[82] Pagano G, Bruno A, Cavallo-Perin P, Cesco L, Imbimbo B. Glucose intolerance after short-term administration of corticosteroids in healthy subjects. Prednisone, deflazacort, and betamethasone. Archives of Internal Medicine. 1989;**149**(5):1098-1101 (Epub May 1, 1989)

[83] Agarwal A, Prasad GV. Post-transplant dyslipidemia: Mechanisms, diagnosis and management. World Journal of Transplantation. 2016;**6**(1):125-134 (Epub Mar 25, 2016)

[84] de Groen PC. Cyclosporine, low-density lipoprotein, and cholesterol. Mayo Clinic Proceedings. 1988;**63**(10):1012-1021 (Epub Oct 1, 1988)

[85] Morrisett JD, Abdel-Fattah G, Hoogeveen R, Mitchell E, Ballantyne CM, Pownall HJ, et al. Effects of sirolimus on plasma lipids, lipoprotein levels, and fatty acid metabolism in renal transplant patients. Journal of Lipid Research. 2002;**43**(8):1170-1180 (Epub Aug 15, 2002)

[86] Holdaas H, Fellstrom B, Jardine AG, Holme I, Nyberg G, Fauchald P, et al. Effect of fluvastatin on cardiac outcomes in renal transplant recipients: A multicentre, randomised, placebo-controlled trial. Lancet. 2003;**361**(9374):2024-2031 (Epub Jun 20, 2003)

[87] Holdaas H, Fellstrom B, Cole E, Nyberg G, Olsson AG, Pedersen TR, et al. Long-term cardiac outcomes in renal transplant recipients receiving fluvastatin: The ALERT extension study. American Journal of Transplantation :

Official Journal of the American Society of Transplantation and the American Society of Transplant Surgeons. 2005;**5**(12):2929-2936 (Epub Nov 24, 2005)

[88] Klein D, Hurley LB, Quesenberry CP Jr, Sidney S. Do protease inhibitors increase the risk for coronary heart disease in patients with HIV-1 infection? Journal of Acquired Immune Deficiency Syndromes. 2002;**30**(5):471-477 (Epub Aug 3, 2002)

[89] Freiberg MS, Chang CC, Kuller LH, Skanderson M, Lowy E, Kraemer KL, et al. HIV infection and the risk of acute myocardial infarction. JAMA Internal Medicine. 2013;**173**(8):614-622 (Epub Mar 6, 2013)

[90] El-Sadr WM, Lundgren J, Neaton JD, Gordin F, Abrams D, Arduino RC, et al. CD4+ count-guided interruption of antiretroviral treatment. The New England Journal of Medicine. 2006;**355**(22):2283-2296 (Epub Dec 1, 2006)

[91] Paisible AL, Chang CC, So-Armah KA, Butt AA, Leaf DA, Budoff M, et al. HIV infection, cardiovascular disease risk factor profile, and risk for acute myocardial infarction. Journal of Acquired Immune Deficiency Syndromes. 2015;**68**(2):209-216 (Epub Jan 15, 2015)

[92] Triant VA. Epidemiology of coronary heart disease in patients with human immunodeficiency virus. Reviews in Cardiovascular Medicine. 2014;**15**(Suppl 1):S1-S8 (Epub Jul 6, 2014)

[93] Rahmanian S, Wewers ME, Koletar S, Reynolds N, Ferketich A, Diaz P. Cigarette smoking in the HIV-infected population. Proceedings of the American Thoracic Society. 2011;**8**(3):313-319 (Epub Jun 10, 2011)

[94] Grinspoon S, Carr A. Cardiovascular risk and body-fat abnormalities in HIV-infected adults. The New England Journal of Medicine. 2005;**352**(1):48-62 (Epub Jan 7, 2005)

[95] Gelpi M, Afzal S, Lundgren J, Ronit A, Roen A, Mocroft A, et al. Higher risk of abdominal obesity, elevated LDL cholesterol and hypertriglyceridemia, but not of hypertension, in people living with HIV: Results from the Copenhagen Comorbidity in HIV Infection (COCOMO) Study. Clinical Infectious Diseases: An Official Publication of the Infectious Diseases Society of America. 1 August 2018;**67**(4):579-586. (Epub Feb 23, 2018)

[96] Micheletti RG, Fishbein GA, Fishbein MC, Singer EJ, Weiss RE, Jeffries RA, et al. Coronary atherosclerotic lesions in human immunodeficiency virus-infected patients: A histopathologic study. Cardiovascular Pathology: The Official Journal of the Society for Cardiovascular Pathology. 2009;**18**(1):28-36 (Epub Apr 12, 2008)

[97] Post WS, Budoff M, Kingsley L, Palella FJ Jr, Witt MD, Li X, et al. Associations between HIV infection and subclinical coronary atherosclerosis. Annals of Internal Medicine. 2014;**160**(7):458-467 (Epub Apr 2, 2014)

[98] Burdo TH, Lo J, Abbara S, Wei J, DeLelys ME, Preffer F, et al. Soluble CD163, a novel marker of activated macrophages, is elevated and associated with noncalcified coronary plaque in HIV-infected patients. The Journal of Infectious Diseases. 2011;**204**(8):1227-1236 (Epub Sep 16, 2011)

[99] Lo J, Abbara S, Shturman L, Soni A, Wei J, Rocha-Filho JA, et al. Increased prevalence of subclinical coronary atherosclerosis detected by coronary computed tomography

angiography in HIV-infected men. AIDS. 2010;**24**(2):243-253 (Epub Dec 10, 2009)

[100] Tawakol A, Lo J, Zanni MV, Marmarelis E, Ihenachor EJ, MacNabb M, et al. Increased arterial inflammation relates to high-risk coronary plaque morphology in HIV-infected patients. Journal of Acquired Immune Deficiency Syndromes. 2014;**66**(2):164-171 (Epub May 16, 2014)

[101] Post WS, George RT, Budoff M. HIV infection and subclinical coronary atherosclerosis. Annals of Internal Medicine. 2014;**161**(12):923-924 (Epub Dec 17, 2014)

[102] Hulten E, Mitchell J, Scally J, Gibbs B, Villines TC. HIV positivity, protease inhibitor exposure and subclinical atherosclerosis: A systematic review and meta-analysis of observational studies. Heart. 2009;**95**(22):1826-1835 (Epub Jul 28, 2009)

[103] Knudsen AD, Gelpi M, Afzal S, Ronit A, Roen A, Mocroft A, et al. Prevalence of peripheral artery disease is higher in persons living with HIV compared to uninfected controls. Journal of Acquired Immune Deficiency Syndromes. 2018 (Epub Jul 10, 2018)

[104] Stanley TL, Grinspoon SK. Body composition and metabolic changes in HIV-infected patients. The Journal of Infectious Diseases. 2012;**205**(Suppl 3): S383-S390 (Epub May 18)

[105] Silverberg MJ, Leyden WA, Xu L, Horberg MA, Chao CR, Towner WJ, et al. Immunodeficiency and risk of myocardial infarction among HIV-positive individuals with access to care. Journal of Acquired Immune Deficiency Syndromes. 2014;**65**(2):160-166 (Epub Jan 21, 2014)

[106] Deeks SG. HIV infection, inflammation, immunosenescence, and aging. Annual Review of Medicine. 2011;**62**:141-155 (Epub Nov 26, 2010)

[107] Chow FC. HIV infection, vascular disease, and stroke. Seminars in Neurology. 2014;**34**(1):35-46 (Epub Apr 10, 2014)

[108] Ganesan A, Crum-Cianflone N, Higgins J, Qin J, Rehm C, Metcalf J, et al. High dose atorvastatin decreases cellular markers of immune activation without affecting HIV-1 RNA levels: Results of a double-blind randomized placebo controlled clinical trial. The Journal of Infectious Diseases. 2011;**203**(6): 756-764 (Epub Feb 18, 2011)

[109] Calza L, Trapani F, Bartoletti M, Manfredi R, Colangeli V, Borderi M, et al. Statin therapy decreases serum levels of high-sensitivity C-reactive protein and tumor necrosis factor-alpha in HIV-infected patients treated with ritonavir-boosted protease inhibitors. HIV Clinical Trials. 2012;**13**(3):153-161 (Epub May 18, 2012)

[110] Holland AT, Palaniappan LP. Problems with the collection and interpretation of Asian-American health data: Omission, aggregation, and extrapolation. Annals of Epidemiology. 2012;**22**(6):397-405 (Epub May 26, 2012)

[111] Miller M, Stone NJ, Ballantyne C, Bittner V, Criqui MH, Ginsberg HN, et al. Triglycerides and cardiovascular disease: A scientific statement from the American Heart Association. Circulation. 2011;**123**(20):2292-2333 (Epub Apr 20, 2011)

[112] Benjamin EJ, Blaha MJ, Chiuve SE, Cushman M, Das SR, Deo R, et al. Heart disease and stroke statistics—2017 update: A report from the American Heart Association. Circulation. 2017;**135**(10):e146-e603 (Epub Jan 27, 2017)

[113] Frank AT, Zhao B, Jose PO, Azar KM, Fortmann SP, Palaniappan LP. Racial/ethnic differences in dyslipidemia patterns. Circulation. 2014;**129**(5):570-579 (Epub Nov 7, 2013)

[114] Anand SS, Yusuf S, Vuksan V, Devanesen S, Teo KK, Montague PA, et al. Differences in risk factors, atherosclerosis, and cardiovascular disease between ethnic groups in Canada: The study of health assessment and risk in ethnic groups (SHARE). Lancet. 2000;**356**(9226):279-284 (Epub Nov 9, 2000)

[115] Goff DC Jr, Bertoni AG, Kramer H, Bonds D, Blumenthal RS, Tsai MY, et al. Dyslipidemia prevalence, treatment, and control in the multi-ethnic study of atherosclerosis (MESA): Gender, ethnicity, and coronary artery calcium. Circulation. 2006;**113**(5):647-656 (Epub Feb 8, 2006)

[116] Rodriguez CJ, Allison M, Daviglus ML, Isasi CR, Keller C, Leira EC, et al. Status of cardiovascular disease and stroke in Hispanics/Latinos in the United States: A science advisory from the American Heart Association. Circulation. 2014;**130**(7):593-625 (Epub Aug 8, 2014)

[117] Hoyert DL. 75 years of mortality in the United States, 1935-2010. NCHS Data Brief. 2012;**88**:1-8 (Epub May 24, 2012)

[118] Marmot MG, Syme SL, Kagan A, Kato H, Cohen JB, Belsky J. Epidemiologic studies of coronary heart disease and stroke in Japanese men living in Japan, Hawaii and California: Prevalence of coronary and hypertensive heart disease and associated risk factors. American Journal of Epidemiology. 1975;**102**(6):514-525 (Epub Dec 1, 1975)

[119] Enas EA, Garg A, Davidson MA, Nair VM, Huet BA, Yusuf S. Coronary heart disease and its risk factors in first-generation immigrant Asian Indians to the United States of America. Indian Heart Journal. 1996;**48**(4): 343-353 (Epub Jul 1, 1996)

[120] Balarajan R. Ethnic differences in mortality from ischaemic heart disease and cerebrovascular disease in England and Wales. British Medical Journal. 1991;**302**(6776):560-564 (Epub Mar 9, 1991)

[121] Gupta M, Brister S. Is south Asian ethnicity an independent cardiovascular risk factor? The Canadian Journal of Cardiology. 2006;**22**(3):193-197 (Epub Mar 8, 2006)

[122] Pencina MJ, Navar-Boggan AM, D'Agostino RB Sr, Williams K, Neely B, Sniderman AD, et al. Application of new cholesterol guidelines to a population-based sample. The New England Journal of Medicine. 2014;**370**(15):1422-1431 (Epub Mar 22, 2014)

[123] Goff DC Jr, Lloyd-Jones DM, Bennett G, Coady S, D'Agostino RB Sr, Gibbons R, et al. ACC/AHA guideline on the assessment of cardiovascular risk: A report of the American College of Cardiology/American Heart Association Task Force on Practice Guidelines. Journal of the American College of Cardiology. 2013, 2014;**63** (25 Pt B):2935-2959 (Epub Nov 19, 2013)

[124] Wilson PW, Pencina MJ. Estimation of risk for initial atherosclerotic cardiovascular disease events: Taking stock and moving forward. Circulation. 2016;**134**(23):1792-1793 (Epub Dec 7, 2016)

[125] Nishizato Y, Ieiri I, Suzuki H, Kimura M, Kawabata K, Hirota T, et al. Polymorphisms of OATP-C (SLC21A6) and OAT3 (SLC22A8) genes: Consequences for pravastatin pharmacokinetics. Clinical Pharmacology and Therapeutics. 2003;**73**(6):554-565 (Epub Jun 18, 2003)

[126] Niemi M. Transporter pharmacogenetics and statin toxicity. Clinical Pharmacology and Therapeutics. 2010;**87**(1):130-133 (Epub Nov 6, 2009)

[127] Pu J, Romanelli R, Zhao B, Azar KM, Hastings KG, Nimbal V, et al. Dyslipidemia in special ethnic populations. Cardiology Clinics. 2015;**33**(2):325-333 (Epub May 6, 2015)

[128] Lee E, Ryan S, Birmingham B, Zalikowski J, March R, Ambrose H, et al. Rosuvastatin pharmacokinetics and pharmacogenetics in white and Asian subjects residing in the same environment. Clinical Pharmacology and Therapeutics. 2005;**78**(4):330-341 (Epub Oct 4, 2005)

[129] Zhang W, Yu BN, He YJ, Fan L, Li Q, Liu ZQ, et al. Role of BCRP 421C>A polymorphism on rosuvastatin pharmacokinetics in healthy Chinese males. Clinica Chimica Acta: International Journal of Clinical Chemistry. 2006;**373**(1-2):99-103 (Epub Jun 21, 2006)

[130] Ho RH, Choi L, Lee W, Mayo G, Schwarz UI, Tirona RG, et al. Effect of drug transporter genotypes on pravastatin disposition in European- and African-American participants. Pharmacogenetics and Genomics. 2007;**17**(8):647-656 (Epub Jul 12, 2007)

[131] HPS2-THRIVE randomized placebo-controlled trial in 25 673 high-risk patients of ER niacin/laropiprant: Trial design, pre-specified muscle and liver outcomes, and reasons for stopping study treatment. European Heart Journal. 2013;**34**(17):1279-1291 (Epub Feb 28, 2013)

[132] Landray MJ, Haynes R, Hopewell JC, Parish S, Aung T, Tomson J, et al. Effects of extended-release niacin with laropiprant in high-risk patients. The New England Journal of Medicine. 2014;**371**(3):203-212 (Epub Jul 12, 2014)

[133] Schoenborn CA, Adams PF, Peregoy JA. Health behaviors of adults: United States, 2008-2010. Vital and health statistics series 10. Data from the National Health Survey. 2013;**257**:1-184 (Epub May 1, 2013)

Chapter 4

Prevalence of Dyslipidemia and Goal Attainment with Lipid-Lowering Therapy: Insights from Thai Multicenter Study and Overview of the Major Guidelines

Songkwan Silaruks, Charn Sriratanasathavorn, Petch Rawdaree, Rapeephon Kunjara-Na-Ayudhaya, Bandit Thinkhamrop and Piyamitr Sritara

Abstract

Background Since the release in Thailand in 2001 of the Third Guidelines by the National Cholesterol Education Program (NCEP) Expert Panel on Detection, Evaluation and Treatment of High Blood Cholesterol in Adults or the Adult Treatment Panel (ATP III), there have been no nationwide studies on the proportion of dyslipidaemic patients who have achieved the low-density lipoprotein cholesterol (LDL-C) goals. The authors therefore aimed to estimate the percentage achievement of LDL-C goals based on the modified NCEP ATP III guidelines in intermediate- to high-risk patients. Methods The authors conducted a hospital-based, cross-sectional, epidemiological survey. Patients (1240) were selected consecutively from 50 hospitals across Thailand. Patients were included if they had been treated with statins for at least 3 months. Results Two-thirds were female, and the mean age was 61.7+69.5 years. The median duration of statin treatment was 21 months. Half (633/1240) of the patients achieved the LDL-C goal levels as defined by the NCEP guidelines (51.1%, 95% CI 48.3% to 53.8%). The very high-risk group had the lowest percentage achievement (11.6%; 95% CI 1.6% to 21.6%), compared with 54.2% (95% CI 50.9% to 57.4%) for the high-risk group and 47.0% (95% CI 41.1% to 52.8%) for the moderate-risk group. More males achieved the LDL-C goals than females (55.6% vs. 48.9%; P = 0.029). Conclusions Overall, 51.1% of the patients with cardiovascular risk, on statins treatment, achieved the NCEP ATP III LDL-C goal levels.

Keywords: dyslipidemia, goal attainment, Thailand

1. Introduction

Dyslipidemia is a major risk factor for the development of atherosclerotic disease. Therefore, lifestyle interventions and pharmacological approaches to decrease cholesterol are widely used in cardiovascular disease prevention. The introduction and widespread use of 3-hydroxy-3-methylglutaryl coenzyme A inhibitors (statins) for individuals at risk of atherosclerotic disease has been an important advance in cardiovascular care [1].

Since 1993, the National Cholesterol Education Program (NCEP) Expert Panel on Detection, Evaluation, and Treatment of High Blood Cholesterol in Adults (Adult Treatment Panel or ATP) has periodically updated the treatment guidelines which identify LDL-C as a cause of CHD and the primary aim for diagnosis and treatment of hypercholesterolaemia [1–3].

In 2001, the recommendations were released in the Third ATP Report (NCEP ATP III) [3] which reaffirmed the risk of CHD from increased LDL-C, the benefit of LDL-C-lowering therapy and maintaining intensive treatment of patients with CHD. The report also added a call for more intensive LDL-C-lowering therapy as the primary aim for patients with a CHD risk equivalent.

There can be no doubt that better control of dyslipidemia, even in subjects whose low-density lipoprotein cholesterol level is not particularly high, has reduced overall event rates. On a background of lifestyle interventions, statins are routinely used to decrease risk along with aspirin and interventions to control hypertension and diabetes. The efficacy of statins in atherosclerotic conditions, particularly in the treatment and prevention of CHD, has been well established [4]. Large-scale, randomized, prospective trials involving patients with CHD have shown that statins reduce the clinical consequences of atherosclerosis, including cardiovascular-related deaths, non-fatal MI and stroke, hospitalization for acute coronary syndrome and heart failure, as well as the need for coronary revascularization [5–7].

2. Clinical practice

Although the guidelines have been widely available, achieving the lower LDL-C goals in practice has been suboptimal. In a US study, only 38% of 4888 patients under primary care in five regions achieved the LDL-C target levels [8]. The respective success rates were 68% and 37% in the low- and high-risk groups. Only 18% of the patients with established CHD with the highest risk of future CHD events achieved the lower LDL-C targets. Another study, based on the records of 461 patients in rural areas, covering all risk levels from four practices, found that only 54% of dyslipidaemic patients achieved the NCEP ATP III goals [9]. In 1998, a survey in Thailand assessing the achievement of LDL-C goals in high-risk patients indicated an unsatisfactorily low percentage of 39.2% [10]. The most recent nationwide survey was conducted between December 2002 and June 2003 [11]. The study involved 1921 patients from 48 hospitals across Thailand. Percentage achievements of LDL-C targets in the CHD and CHD equivalents, high-, and low-risk group were 34.6, 56.4 and 76.8%, respectively [11]. In 2004, several changes were made to the guideline, released as the Modified NCEP ATP III in that year [12]. There has, however, been no recent nationwide study in Thailand investigating the proportion of dyslipidemia patients who have achieved the updated LDL-C goals.

3. Clinical practice in Thailand

In our study [13], we conducted a hospital-based, cross-sectional, epidemiological survey and retrospective chart review, in both secondary and tertiary care across Thailand. Our study aimed to estimate the percentage of LDL-C goals achievement based on the NCEP ATP III guidelines in intermediate- to high-risk patients receiving statins for at least 3 months in clinical practice in Thailand. The data collection was conducted at the selected hospitals between March and July 2008. The primary outcome of this study was the percentage of dyslipidaemic patients on lipid-lowering therapy who had achieved their respective LDL-C target levels as defined by the NCEP ATP III guidelines.

3.1 Number of patients and participating hospitals

There are 95 secondary- and tertiary-care hospitals across Thailand, 50 (52.6%) of which were selected for the study. The number of selected hospitals in each region was proportional to the total number of eligible hospitals in each region (i.e., the North, the Northeast, the South and Central). A total of 1730 patients attending OPD clinics were screened by interviews, and 167 (9.6%) were excluded: 161 not currently treated with statin, five not consented and one not within 20–80 years of age. After the chart review was conducted, a further 323 (20.7%) cases were excluded: 216 treated <3 months before lipid profile became available, 32 lipid profile not available and 75 having not received the same statin before lipid profile became available.

The duration of statin treatment prior to the date of the most recent lipid profile ranged between 3 and 191 months (median 21 months), which represented the period of statin treatment at the time of assessing the treatment outcome.

The high-risk group accounted for the largest number of patients, followed by moderate- and high-risk patient types. The mean age was 61.7 ± 9.5 years, and approximately two-thirds were female. The mean age of each risk group was similar. Overall, the majority of males at risk (94%) were 45 years of age or higher. A similar percentage was seen in each risk group. For females at risk, about three-quarters were aged 55 years or older. Most common cardiovascular risks were diabetes mellitus (66.1%) and hypertension (57.6%).

3.2 Percentage achievement of LDL-C goals for all patients

Among the 1240 patients, 633 achieved the lower LDL-C goals as defined by the NCEP ATP III guidelines (51.1%; 95% CI 48.3% to 53.8%) (**Table 1**). The very high-risk group had the lowest achievement level at about one tenth. The achievement rate varies among regions where the highest achievement rate was 57.4% in the central area, and the lowest achievement rate was 42.6% in the eastern part of the country. On average, the very high-risk patients were about half, 49.7%, to reach the LDL-C target goal.

Patient groups*	Total	Achieved goals	Percentage	95% CI	Mean percentage† to target LDL-C
Very high risk	43	5	11.6	1.6 to 21.6	49.7
High risk	914	495	54.2	50.9 to 57.4	31.8
Moderate risk	283	133	47.0	41.1 to 52.8	9.9
Overall	1240	633	51.1	48.3 to 53.8	27.5

**Very high risk (LDL-C < 70 mg/dl); high risk (LDL-C < 100 mg/dl); moderate risk (LDL-C < 130 mg/dl).*
†Calculated based on the percentage difference between LDL-C level and the target goal among patients who did not achieve the LDL-C target.

Table 1.
Percentage and 95% CIs of low-density lipoprotein cholesterol (LDL-C) achievement goals by patient group.

Males had a statistically higher percentage achievement of the lower LDL-C goals than females (p = 0.024) (**Table 1**). The duration of statin treatment and the statin use, either alone or combined with other regimens, had a similar percentage achievement of lower LDL-C goals.

The final number of subjects included in the analysis was 1240. Initially, the calculated sample size was 1260, of which 20 (1.8%) patients had a statin treatment of <3 months. These were identified after enrolment and excluded from the analysis. This elimination did not, however, affect the study findings, that is, the percentage achievement of LDL-C goals was 52.5% when they were included, compared with 51.1% when they were excluded.

We, thus, included only patients who had been treated for at least 3 months with no maximum limit of treatment duration. The results in **Table 2** indeed suggest that the duration of statin treatment had no effect on the percentage achievement of LDL-C goals, which was about 51% for every interval of 12 months (p = 0.975).

Selected factors	No	Percentage achievement	p Value
Gender			0.029
Male	417	55.4	
Female	823	48.9	
Male by age (years) at risk			0.750
≥45	394	55.6	
<45	23	52.2	
Female by age (years) at risk			0.057
≥55 of age	623	50.7	
<55	200	43.0	
Duration (months) of statin treatment			0.997
3–6	136	50.7	
7–12	245	51.0	
13–24	349	50.4	
25–36	235	51.9	
≥37	275	51.3	
Statins received			0.842
Statins only	1156	51.1	
Statins with other lipid-lowering drugs	84	50.0	
Field of expertise of attending physicians			0.360
Internal medicine	1227	51.2	
Non-internal medicine	13	38.5	
Field of expertise of attending physicians who were in internal medicine			0.598
General	1029	51.2	
Cardiologist	128	53.9	
Endocrinologist, nephrologists or neurologist	67	46.3	

Table 2.
Percentage low-density lipoprotein cholesterol achievement goals by selected factors.

However, there are numerous factors which may confound the goal achievement, including statin dose, potency of statin, culture, socio-economic status, healthcare policy, concomitant medications, etc. Also, the selection bias from selected study sites, which were from diabetes and hypertension clinics even we tried to do the study in various parts of the country. This leads to a higher proportion of high-risk group than general populations.

Our study was based on the availability of lipid profiles of patients measured on request, as per real-life clinical practice; however, there were no significant differences between the percentage achievement of LDL-C goals among patients whose lipid profile was assessed before or after the median of 5.5 months prior to the survey date. This result might indicate that LDL-C levels were underutilized to adjust the treatment.

In our study, the percentage of lowered LDL-C according to goal levels, as defined by NCEP ATP III guidelines, among the high-cardiovascular-risk group, was 51.1% compared with 39.2% in a 1997–1998 study [10] and 34.6% in the 2002–2003 study [14]. The higher percentage found in our study could be due to various reasons: (1) we included only patients who used statins and not any other lipid-lowering agent alone; (2) there has been an increasing focus on the benefits of intensive cholesterol reduction; (3) new and more efficacious statins have been developed; (4) 95% of the patients in our study were attended by specialists who might be more likely to adhere to the guidelines; and (5) two-thirds of the patients in our study were females, who might have had a greater rate of compliance to the treatment or might have had a greater response to therapy than males, although there are few data to support this. As with other studies, our study found that the lowest percentage of achieving the recommended LDL-C target was in the very high-risk group [10, 14].

A number of aspects of our study can be considered strengths. First, the case selection was unbiased, as it was carried out consecutively and independent of the attending physicians. Second, we covered a large number (52.6%) of secondary- and tertiary-care hospitals across the country. Third, almost all of the studied patients (99.0%) were attended by an internal medicine, specialist, particularly the very high-risk and high-risk patients. Finally, our study represented real-life, clinical settings in Thailand, so the percentage achievement of LDL-C goals may represent clinical practice.

In summary, our study demonstrated that 51.1% of patients with cardiovascular risk on statin treatment achieved the LDL-C goal levels defined by the NCEP ATP III guidelines. We suggest that patients with a high CHD risk should be targeted for more aggressive lipid-lowering management. National campaigns to increase the awareness among both physicians and patients of the importance of achieving the LDL-C goals are needed to optimize the prevention of cardiovascular events and to further reduce the burden of cardiovascular diseases. Further investigation is needed to understand the reasons for patients not achieving lower LDL-C levels.

4. Clinical implications in real world practice

Despite the >50% decrease in age-adjusted cardiovascular mortality over the past several decades, atherosclerotic disease is still the leading cause of morbidity and mortality. Moreover, cardiovascular disease accounts for more than half of all non-communicable diseases and has become the leading cause of death worldwide, a fact affirmed by the World Health Organization [15]. Large cohort studies dating back to the Framingham Heart Study have identified cholesterol as a modifiable risk factor, which can be treated with lifestyle and pharmacological interventions

[16]. Total cholesterol levels have decreased in high-income countries over the past 2 decades by 8–10% on average. Some countries with the highest levels were able to decrease levels more than this with targeted societal interventions, leading directly to dramatic decreases in event rates. As part of the United Nations declaration on non-communicable diseases, with a goal of reducing premature death by 25%, their target is a 20% relative reduction in high total cholesterol by 2025. To be truly effective, the treatment of dyslipidemia needs to be incorporated into a comprehensive plan of global risk reduction for patients at risk. This will involve lifestyle modification, policy change, and pharmacotherapy.

5. Similarities and differences in dyslipidemia guidelines

New dyslipidemia guidelines were released by the European Society of Cardiology (ESC)/European Atherosclerosis Society (EAS) in 2011 [17], the CCS in 2012 [18], the International Atherosclerosis Society [19], and the American College of Cardiology (ACC)/American Heart Association (AHA), both in 2013 [20]. All are similar in many respects, yet have some key differences that are worthy of discussion. The 2012 CCS guidelines recommended risk stratification using the total cardiovascular disease **F**ramingham **R**isk **S**core (FRS) [21], advocated the use of low-density lipoprotein cholesterol (LDL-C) thresholds for the initiation of treatment in low- and intermediate-risk subjects and expanded the phenotype of high-risk subjects to include subjects with atherosclerosis, most patients with diabetes, high-risk hypertension (per **A**nglo-**S**candinavian **C**ardiac **O**utcomes **T**rial [ASCOT] inclusion criteria) [22] and predialysis chronic kidney disease (CKD). LDL-C continues to be used as the atherogenic metric, but now non-high-density lipoprotein cholesterol (HDL-C) and apolipoprotein B (apo B) could be measured as alternatives, especially under circumstances when LDL-C calculations are known to be erroneous. When treatment is initiated, LDL-C (<2.0 mmol/L or 50% reduction) continues to be the primary target of therapy. The CCS guidelines have been harmonized with other relevant Canadian guidelines as part of the Canadian Cardiovascular Harmonization National Guidelines Endeavor (C-CHANGE) initiative [23] (**Table 3**).

The ESC/EAS guidelines was a comprehensive document that encouraged the use of the **S**ystematic **Co**ronary **R**isk **E**valuation (SCORE) total cardiovascular mortality [24].

Calibrated for high- or low-risk countries in Europe. Of note, the SCORE risk assessment is also based on the Framingham risk equation. LDL-C thresholds were suggested with non-HDL-C or apo B as alternatives. The European guidelines also recognized CKD as very high-risk equivalent. Target levels of LDL-C were recommended but unlike the CCS guidelines, the goals were different between those at very high risk (<1.8 mmol/L) compared with those at high risk (<2.5 mmol/L) or intermediate risk (<3.0 mmol/L).

The International Atherosclerosis Society panel decided to recommend lifetime cardiovascular risk based on 4 different tools depending on ethnicity. They favored non-HDL-C as the primary atherogenic metric for risk determination, with LDL-C as a secondary measure. Optimal levels were defined based on criteria from Adult Treatment Panel-III (ATP-III), but did not recommend treatment targets. The intensity of statin therapy should be adjusted according to overall lifetime risk and practitioner practice.

The ACC/AHA guidelines were the latest to be released and created the most controversy [20]. A major novel aspect of these guidelines was the recommendation to calculate risk using the newly developed Pooled Cohort Equation. This approach

DOI: http://dx.doi.org/10.5772/intechopen.82355

Guidelines	Year	Major features	Limitations
European Society of Cardiology (ESC)/European Atherosclerosis Society (EAS) in 2011 [17]	2011	Comprehensive document that encouraged the use of the Systematic Coronary Risk Evaluation (SCORE) total cardiovascular mortality 10 calibrated for high- or low-risk countries in Europe. Also recognized CKD as very high-risk equivalent	Target levels of LDL-C were recommended but unlike the CCS guidelines, the goals were different between those at very high risk (<1.8 mmol/L) compared with those at high risk (<2.5 mmol/L) or intermediate risk (<3.0 mmol/L)
Canadian Cardiovascular Society Guidelines (CCS) 2012 [18]	2012	Risk stratification using the total cardiovascular disease Framingham Risk Score (FRS), use of LDL-C thresholds for the initiation of treatment in low- and intermediate-risk subjects and expanded the phenotype of high-risk subjects to include subjects with atherosclerosis, most patients with diabetes, high-risk hypertension	LDL-C continues to be used as the atherogenic metric, but non-high-density lipoprotein cholesterol (HDL-C) and apolipoprotein B (apo B) could be measured as alternatives, especially under circumstances when LDL-C calculations are known to be erroneous
International Atherosclerosis Society [19]	2013	Recommend lifetime cardiovascular risk based on 4 different tools depending on ethnicity. They favored non-HDL-C as the primary atherogenic metric for risk determination, with LDL-C as a secondary measure. Optimal levels were defined based on criteria from Adult Treatment Panel-III (ATP-III)	Not recommend treatment targets. The intensity of statin therapy should be adjusted according to overall lifetime risk and practitioner practice.
American College of Cardiology (ACC)/ American Heart Association (AHA) [20]	2013	Recommendation to calculate risk using the newly developed Pooled Cohort Equation. No recommendation for treating to any specific target. "Fire and forget" approach	Created the most controversy. Novel aspect was the recommendation to calculate risk using the newly developed Pooled Cohort Equation. The new risk engine tended to overestimate events.

Table 3.
Similarities and differences in dyslipidemia guidelines.

represents a departure from the use of the FRS, used for decades. Of the 4 groups targeted for statin-based therapy, 3 were the same as the CCS guidelines. These include subjects with: (1) clinical evidence of atherosclerosis; (2) most subjects with diabetes; and (3) individuals with LDL-C ≥5.0 mmol/L. The fourth group includes subjects with a 10-year risk of total atherosclerotic events calculated using the Pooled Cohort Equation of ≥7.5% [25, 26]. There was no specific recommendation for CKD and other populations such as genetic dyslipidemia or high-risk hypertension. An additional novel aspect of these guidelines was the lack of specific targets of therapy. Although these guidelines recommend the use of high- or moderate-intensity statin regimens based on level of risk and anticipate a 50% LDL-C decrease with high-intensity statin therapy, there is no recommendation for treating to any specific target. Therefore, lipid measurements after initiation of statin therapy are recommended, primarily to ensure adherence.

6. The elimination of atherogenic lipoprotein targets

The new ACC/AHA guidelines were distinctly different from most previous recommendations in that they have discarded specific LDL-C (or alternative) targets when subjects are initiated with therapy. The rationale for this change was that no previous randomized trial specifically addressed whether a particular level produced greater event reduction. Second, by eliminating targets it was believed that primary care treatment would be more straightforward and easier to implement. Third, having targets potentially promotes combination therapy, for which there is currently no good evidence from randomized trials. This is supported by data from meta-analysis of trials of fibrate therapy, **A**therothrombosis **I**ntervention in **M**etabolic Syndrome with Low **HDL**/High triglycerides and **I**mpact on **G**lobal **H**ealth Outcomes (AIM-HIGH) and **H**eart **P**rotection **S**tudy **2**: **T**reatment of **HDL** to **R**educe the **I**ncidence of **V**ascular **E**vents (HPS2-THRIVE) [27–29].When using combination therapy one must be aware that the addition of either fibrates or niacin to statin therapy may increase the risk of myositis. The increased risk of myositis is greatest when gemfibrozil is used in combination with statins. Fenofibrate has a much more modest risk and the FDA approved the use of fenofibrate in combination with moderate doses of statins. The increased risk with niacin appears to be modest. In the AIM-HIGH trial the risk of myositis was not increased in patients on the combination of Niaspan and statin, whereas in the HPS2-Thrive trial myopathy was increased in the group treated with the combination of niacin and statin. The absolute risks of combination therapy are relatively modest if patients are carefully selected; in many patients at high risk for cardiovascular disease combination therapy may be appropriate. As with many decisions in medicine one needs to balance the benefits of therapy with the risks of therapy and determine for the individual patient the best approach. In deciding to use combination therapy a key focus is the non-HDL-C level. When the LDL is at goal but the non-HDL-C is still markedly above goal it may be appropriate to resort to combination therapy in patients at high risk.

Although this interpretation is literally correct, it fails to recognize several issues in the history of statin trials: the initial trials were as much studies of the lipid hypothesis as they were trials of statins. Thus, the first trials were in patients with the highest risk and highest cholesterol levels but at a time when only moderately potent statins were available, hence the use of the highest dose feasible. Because success was shown, and as more potent statins became available, ethical considerations mandated that research subjects had to have lower and lower risk and lower and lower cholesterol levels, again promoting use of the highest available dose. The latter was also influenced by a need to ensure simplicity in large trials and, to some extent, by marketing designed to promote drug potency differences. There are also 5 trials of higher vs. lower potency statins, which show consistent improvement in outcomes with the higher potency statin. The lowest risk cohort studied to date in the **J**ustification for the **U**se of Statins in **P**revention: An **I**ntervention **T**rial **E**valuating **R**osuvastatin (JUPITER) study reaped comparable benefit using the most potent statin currently available. Remarkably, no lower limit of achieved LDL-C beyond which benefit is accrued has yet been shown. The CCS dyslipidemia guideline primary panel reviewed these issues in early 2014 and recommended that until further evidence was available, we would continue to support the use of targets. Although it is certainly true that randomized trials have generally used a single statin dose approach, as opposed to a target LDL-C level, the epidemiology suggesting that lower levels of achieved LDL-C result in less events is rather compelling. Also, regression studies with intravascular ultrasound demonstrate a linear relationship between LDL-C and the amount of regression [30]. The crossing point for regression tends to occur at an LDL-C of around 2 mmol/L or a 50% reduction. A very recent meta-analysis used individual patient data from 8 statin trials [31]. Using a fixed dose of statin, there was a very large inter-individual variation in LDL-C reduction with statins. In addition, more than 40% of subjects did not achieve targets of <1.8 mmol/L with a fixed statin dose. Those who achieved very low levels of LDL-C had a lower event rate than those who achieved modest levels. The same trend was seen for non-HDL-C and apo B.

We will be able to test the "lower is better" hypothesis at very low levels of LDL-C when the results of ongoing trials using nonstatins (e.g., inhibitors of cholesterol absorption, proprotein convertase subtisilin/kexin type 9 (PCSK9) and cholesterol ester transfer protein (CETP) are well established and widely applicable to practitioners.

The ACC/AHA guidelines would appear at first blush to support a "fire and forget" approach. The text and algorithms do, however, suggest that measuring LDL-C after statin initiation is reasonable to help assess compliance and to ensure achievement of an expected percentage of decrease of LDL-C. Compliance and adherence are important issues with statin therapy [32] and beyond the scope of this review, but are certainly another practical reason that the CCS guidelines panel continues to recommend targets. Additionally, the text and algorithms of the ACC/AHA guidelines promote LDL-C measurement to ensure achievement of the expected response to moderate- and high-intensity statin dose choices and, when not achieved or in the face of statin intolerance, support dose escalation or addition of secondary, non-statin drugs.

The new ACC/AHA guidelines have generated considerable debate and confusion in the medical literature about the specifics of risk assessment and treatment of dyslipidemia in cardiovascular disease prevention. It is healthy to accept that there are different approaches to screening and management, because of the lack of decisive evidence in certain domains. The discussion should be used to highlight the need to address outstanding questions in the future. However, in the interim, our patients can be very well managed with existing guidelines that are updated on an ongoing basis when new knowledge is generated. A guidelines-based approach to screening, treatment, and compliance should continue to be the standard for all of our at-risk patients.

In conclusion, the National Guideline campaigns to increase the awareness among both physicians and patients of the importance of achieving the LDL-C goals are needed to optimize the prevention of cardiovascular events and to further reduce the burden of cardiovascular diseases.

Author details

Songkwan Silaruks[1*], Charn Sriratanasathavorn[2], Petch Rawdaree[3], Rapeephon Kunjara-Na-Ayudhaya[4], Bandit Thinkhamrop[5] and Piyamitr Sritara[6]

1 Department of Medicine, Khon Kaen University, Khon Kaen, Thailand

2 Her Majesty's Cardiac Center, Department of Medicine, Siriraj Hospital, Mahidol University, Bangkok, Thailand

3 Endocrinology Unit, BMA Medical College, Vajira Hospital, Thailand

4 Vichaiyut Hospital, Thailand

5 Department of Biostatistics and Demography, Khon Kaen University, Khon Kaen, Thailand

6 Department of Medicine, Ramathibodi Hospital, Mahidol University, Bangkok, Thailand

*Address all correspondence to: sonsil@kku.ac.th

References

[1] Anon. Summary of the second report of the national cholesterol education program (NCEP) expert panel on detection, evaluation, and treatment of high blood cholesterol in adults (adult treatment panel II). JAMA. 1993;**269**:3015-3023

[2] Anon. National cholesterol education program. Second report of the expert panel on detection, evaluation, and treatment of high blood cholesterol in adults (adult treatment panel II). Circulation. 1994;**89**:1333-1445. [PubMed]

[3] Expert Panel on Detection, Evaluation, and Treatment of High Blood Cholesterol in Adults. Executive summary of the third report of the National Cholesterol Education Program (NCEP) expert panel on detection, evaluation, and treatment of high blood cholesterol in adults (adult treatment panel III). JAMA. 2001;**285**:2486-2497

[4] Anderson TJ, Mancini GB, Genest J Jr, Gregoire J, Lonn EM, Hegele RA. The new dyslipidemia guidelines: What is the debate? The Canadian Journal of Cardiology. 2015;**31**(5):605-612. DOI: 10.1016/j.cjca.2014.11.007

[5] Baigent C, Keech A, Kearney PM, et al. Efficacy and safety of cholesterol-lowering treatment: Prospective meta-analysis of data from 90,056 participants in 14 randomised trials of statins. Lancet. 2005;**366**:1267-1278. [PubMed]

[6] LaRosa JC, Grundy SM, Waters DD, et al. Intensive lipid lowering with atorvastatin in patients with stable coronary disease. The New England Journal of Medicine. 2005;**352**: 1425-1435. [PubMed]

[7] Rosenson R. Statins: Can the new generation make an impression? Expert Opinion on Emerging Drugs. 2004;**9**:269-279. [PubMed]

[8] Pearson TA, Laurora I, Chu H, et al. The lipid treatment assessment project (L-TAP): A multicenter survey to evaluate the percentages of dyslipidemic patients receiving lipid-lowering therapy and achieving low-density lipoprotein cholesterol goals. Archives of Internal Medicine. 2000;**160**:459-467

[9] Qayyum R, Chattha AA, Bhullar N, et al. Achievement of national cholesterol education program goals by patients with dyslipidemia in rural ambulatory care settings. Preventive Cardiology. 2006;**9**:192-197

[10] Nitiyanant W, Ngamukos P, Koanantakul B. Lipid treatment assessment project (L-TAP) in Thailand. Internal Medical Journal of Thailand. 2001;**17**:246-252

[11] Nitiyanant Ws P, Deerochanawong C. The Lipid Treatment Assessment Project II (L-TAP II) in Thailand. L-TAP II in Thailand Free Paper and Poster presented at 15th ASEAN Congress of Cardiology (ACC). Pattaya, Thailand: The 15th ASEAN Congress of Cardiology (ACC); 2004

[12] Johnson LW, Weinstock RS. The metabolic syndrome: Concepts and controversy. Mayo Clinic Proceedings. 2006;**81**:1615-1620

[13] Silaruks S, Sriratanasathavorn C, Rawdaree P, Na-Ayudhaya K, Thinkhamrop B, Sritara P. Lipid-lowering therapy using statins in patients with cardiovascular risk in clinical practice in Thailand. Heart Asia. 2011;**3**(1):99-103

[14] Nitiyanant W, Sritara P, Deerochanawong C, et al. Lipid treatment assessment project II in Thailand (LTAP-II Thailand). Journal of the Medical Association of Thailand. 2008;**91**:836-845

[15] Laslett LJ, Alagona P Jr, Clark BA 3rd, et al. Journal of the American College of Cardiology. 2012;**60**:S1-S49

[16] Wilson PW, D'Agostino RB, Levy D, et al. Prediction of coronary heart disease using risk factor categories. Circulation. 1998;**97**:1837-1847

[17] European Association for Cardiovascular Prevention and Rehabilitation, Reiner Z, Catapano AL, et al. European Heart Journal. 2011;**32**:1769-1818

[18] Anderson TJ, Gregoire J, Hegele RA, et al. 2012 update of the Canadian cardiovascular society guidelines for the diagnosis and treatment of dyslipidemia for the prevention of cardiovascular disease in the adult. The Canadian Journal of Cardiology. 2013;**29**:151-167

[19] Expert Dyslipidemia Panel of the International Atherosclerosis Society Panel members. An international atherosclerosis society position paper: Global recommendations for the management of dyslipidemia–full report. Journal of Clinical Lipidology. 2014;**8**:29-60

[20] Stone NJ, Robinson J, Lichtenstein AH, et al. 2013 ACC/AHA guideline on the treatment of blood cholesterol to reduce atherosclerotic cardiovascular risk in adults: A report of the American College of Cardiology/American Heart Association task force on practice guidelines. [erratum in 2014;63:3024-5]. Journal of the American College of Cardiology. 2013;**63**:2889-2934

[21] D'Agostino RB Sr, Vasan RS, Pencina MJ, et al. General cardiovascular risk profile for use in primary care: The Framingham heart study. Circulation. 2008;**117**:743-753

[22] Sever PS, Dahlof B, Poulter NR, et al. Prevention of coronary and stroke events with atorvastatin in hypertensive patients who have average or lower-than-average cholesterol concentrations, in the anglo-scandinavian cardiac outcomes trial–lipid lowering arm (ASCOT-LLA): A multicentre randomised controlled trial. Lancet. 2003;**361**:1149-1158

[23] Tobe SW, Stone JA, Brouwers M, et al. Harmonization of guidelines for the prevention and treatment of cardiovascular disease: The C-CHANGE initiative. CMAJ. 2011;**183**:E1135-E1150

[24] Conroy RM, Pyorala K, Fitzgerald AP, et al. Estimation of ten-year risk of fatal cardiovascular disease in Europe: The SCORE project. European Heart Journal. 2003;**24**:987-1003

[25] Goff DC Jr, Lloyd-Jones DM, Bennett G, et al. Circulation. 2013;**129**(25 suppl 2):S49-S73

[26] Ridker PM, Cook Statins NR. New American guidelines for prevention of cardiovascular disease. Lancet. 2013;**382**:1762-1765

[27] AIM-HIGH Investigators, Boden WE, Probstfield JL, et al. Niacin in patients with low HDL cholesterol levels receiving intensive statin therapy. The New England Journal of Medicine. 2011;**365**:2255-2267

[28] HPS2-THRIVE Collaborative Group, Landray MJ, Haynes R, et al. The New England Journal of Medicine. 2014;**371**:203-212

[29] Cholesterol Treatment Trialists' (CTT) Collaborators, Mihaylova B, Emberson J, et al. The effects of lowering LDL cholesterol with statin therapy in people at low risk of vascular disease: Meta-analysis of individual data from 27 randomised trials. Lancet, 2012;**380**:581-590

[30] Ballantyne M, Raichlen JS, Nicholls SJ, et al. Effect of rosuvastatin therapy on coronary artery stenoses assessed by quantitative coronary

angiography: A study to evaluate the effect of rosuvastatin on intravascular ultrasound-derived coronary atheroma burden. Circulation. 2008;**117**:2458-2466

[31] Boekholdt SM, Hovingh GK, Mora S, et al. Very low levels of atherogenic lipoproteins and the risk for cardiovascular events: A meta-analysis of statin trials. Journal of the American College of Cardiology. 2014;**64**:485-494

[32] Ben-Yehuda AN. DeMariaLDL-cholesterol targets after the ACC/AHA 2013 guidelines: Evidence that lower is better? Journal of the American College of Cardiology. 2014;**64**:495-497

Chapter 5

Postprandial Lipemia as Cardiovascular Disease Risk Factor

Neil Francis Amba and Leilani B. Mercado-Asis

Abstract

Postprandial lipemia (PPL) is characterized by prolonged and increased levels of lipids especially triglycerides (TG) and triglyceride-rich lipoprotein levels after a meal. There are an increasing number of evidence that postprandial lipemia is a significant risk factor for cardiovascular disease because of its causative role in atherosclerosis and endothelial dysfunction. This has serious implications because common dietary patterns are characterized by high fat content and meal consumption; hence, most will be in a postprandial state resulting to frequent and prolonged exposure to high lipid levels. The review will present the current evidences for the role of postprandial lipemia as a risk factor for cardiovascular disease and its association with other cardiovascular risk factors, namely, diabetes and obesity. We will also present recommendations on the diagnosis and management of postprandial lipemia.

Keywords: postprandial lipemia, postprandial dyslipidemia, endothelial dysfunction, hypertriglyceridemia

1. Lipoprotein metabolism

Lipoproteins are responsible for the distribution of cholesterol and triglyceride from the intestine and liver to peripheral cells. The process of lipoprotein distribution and metabolism is highly related to energy metabolism and the feed-fast cycle. Triglycerides (TG) are synthesized from dietary free fatty acids and glycerol in enterocytes. They are assembled together with phospholipids and cholesterol with apolipoproteins, mainly apoB-48 into chylomicron particles (apo A, C, E also present). These TG-rich particles enter the plasma via the intestinal lymph. Chylomicrons are then transported to peripheral cells where the enzyme lipoprotein lipase (LPL) hydrolyses their triglyceride content, releasing free fatty acids to be used by peripheral cells. The resulting chylomicron remnants are smaller and denser and are removed in the circulation by binding of the surface apo E to the LDL receptor or LDL receptor-related protein (LRP) [1]. Please also refer to the introductory chapter of this book for detailed and illustrated review of lipoprotein metabolism.

In the liver, synthesized TGs are released to the circulation by the very low-density lipoprotein (VLDL) particles. VLDL particles are TG-rich and, mainly, apo B-100-containing particles (apo A, C, E also present). VLDL synthesis takes place

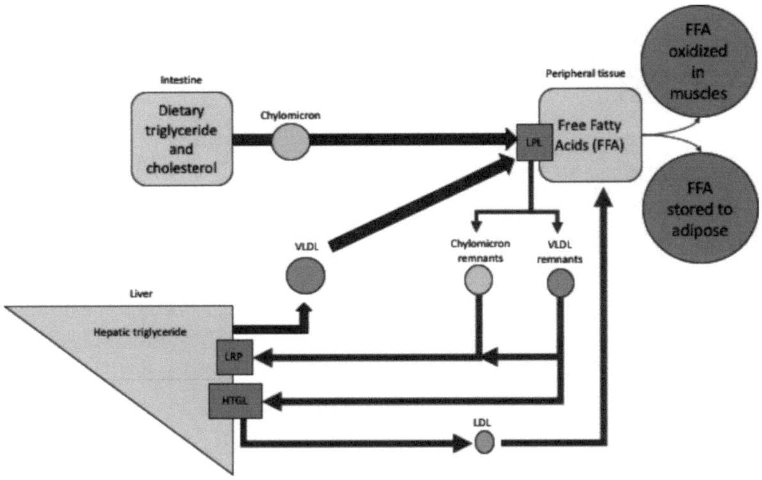

Figure 1.
Lipoprotein metabolism overview. Dietary TG transported via chylomicrons and hepatic TG transported via VLDL are delivered to peripheral tissue and acted upon by lipoprotein lipase to liberate fatty acids for energy fuel, cellular synthesis, or fat storage. Chylomicron and VLDL remnants are taken up by the liver. VLDL remnants can be further hydrolyzed by HTGL to form LDL particles.

during fasting and prandial state. Once delivered to peripheral tissues, the TG contents are hydrolyzed to free fatty acids by LPL, similar to that of chylomicrons. VLDL remnants, also called intermediate-density lipoproteins (IDL), are taken up by the liver via apo E binding to LDL receptor or converted to LDL by removal of TG content by the hepatic triglyceride lipase (HTGL) enzyme. The removal of TG renders the particles smaller allowing better vascular penetration, hence increasing atherogenicity [2].

The cholesterol ester transfer protein (CETP) facilitates the transfer of cholesteryl esters from high-density lipoproteins (HDL) particles to VLDL in exchange for TGs. Cholesteryl ester-enriched particles are better substrates for HTGL allowing greater decrease in size of the particle, creating small dense (sd) LDL. Small, dense LDL are more atherogenic due to their smaller size as they readily enter the subendothelial space [1].

Chylomicrons, VLDL, and their respective remnants (remnant lipoproteins (RLP)) are termed triacylglycerol-rich lipoproteins (TRL) (**Figure 1**).

2. Lipid profile in the postprandial state

The plasma lipid levels normally fluctuate during the day, in response to food intake. TG levels vary more considerably compared to LDL and HDL cholesterol levels. Nowadays, the common dietary habit is characterized by high fat contents and high frequency of meals; hence, most individuals will be in a nonfasting state. Because of the evidence of association of nonfasting lipid levels as a risk factor for CVD, it is important to analyze postprandial lipoprotein physiology and metabolism [2].

In a study by Stanhope et al., it has been found that TG levels are significantly elevated during the day in association to food intake. When fructose was administered, there was significant increase in TG compared with the regular meal. Plasma cholesterol levels did not significantly change during the day [3]. In our previous studies, we were able to demonstrate the pattern of postprandial lipid rise. We have found that there was significant increase in the levels for total cholesterol, triglycerides, and HDL with peaking at the 4th–5th hour after a fatty meal [4]. The postprandial increase in TG is again demonstrated in another study by our group and has shown to be similar with VLDL postprandial increase beginning 4 hours after breakfast and sustained until 9–10 hours after [5]. In one of our trials, similar patterns of postprandial increase in TC, TG, and HDL were demonstrated with peaking at the 4th–5th hour and with noted decline at the 5th–6th hour [6]. None of our studies have demonstrated any pattern of postprandial rise for LDL.

The postprandial period is characterized by an increase in atherogenic lipoprotein particles. These are the TRLs including chylomicrons, VLDL, and their remnant particles. Their levels are affected by multiple individual and environmental factors, including sex, age, body mass index, physical activity, and smoking, and by the amount and type of dietary fat in a meal [7].

In the study by Cohn et al., they have shown that there may be more than one peak in postprandial TG concentration, that the magnitude of postprandial rise is dependent on age and gender, that postprandial plasma cholesterol concentration can increase or remain at baseline, and that postprandial cholesterolemia is inversely correlated with fasting HDL levels [8].

The postprandial lipid response has been shown to be modified by polymorphisms within the genes for apo A-I, E, B, C-I, C-III, A-IV, and A-V, LPL, hepatic lipase, fatty acid-binding protein-2, the fatty acid transport proteins, microsomal triglyceride transfer protein, and scavenger receptor class B Type I [9].

3. Postprandial lipemia in diabetes

Diabetes is associated with premature atherosclerosis and cardiovascular disease, and this may be contributed to diabetic dyslipidemia. Diabetes is characterized by multiple lipoprotein metabolism abnormalities that promote atherogenesis. The common lipid abnormality in diabetes includes hypertriglyceridemia, low HDL, and increase in small, dense LDL (sdLDL) levels. In a study by Shukla that investigated the postprandial response of type 2 DM patients after a standard fat challenge, it has been found that compared to normal controls, DM patients have significantly higher postprandial triglyceride levels despite having similar fasting levels. No significant difference in postprandial HDL levels was seen when adjusted to fasting levels [10].

The abnormalities in lipids among diabetics are secondary to multiple metabolic derangement that characterizes diabetes. For example, it has also been found that intestinal lipoprotein metabolism among diabetics is altered with increased lipoprotein production that prolongs postprandial lipemia [11].

In our clinic-based retrospective study, we have found that HbA1c has strong positive correlation with postprandial TG, while the 2-hour plasma glucose has moderate positive correlation. These significant correlations of postprandial lipemia with glycemic control and postprandial glycemia suggest that despite optimal fasting lipid levels, poor glycemic control is still associated with elevation of postprandial lipids, specifically postprandial triglycerides [12]. Similarly, Nakamura et al. have demonstrated that insulin resistance is closely related to postprandial hyperlipidemia among type 2 DM patients with CAD. Specifically, they have found that the 6th hour postprandial TG and remnant-like particle cholesterol were significantly higher among type 2 DM subjects and that plasma insulin levels and insulin resistance index were correlated with serum TG and RLP-C levels [13]. In addition, it has been shown in an animal study that postprandial hypertriglyceridemia predicts the development of insulin resistance, glucose intolerance, and type 2 DM [14]. However, evidence is still lacking.

Although it has been shown that glycemia is correlated with postprandial dyslipidemia, there are evidences that even with good glycemic control, diabetes is still associated with postprandial dyslipidemia. Rivellese et al. have demonstrated that subjects with type 2 DM with good glucose control and optimal fasting triglyceride levels still presented with abnormal plasma lipid response after a standard mixed meal. In particular, large VLDL and chylomicron remnants were shown to be elevated postprandially [15].

4. Postprandial lipemia and obesity

Obesity is a global epidemic affecting both children and adults. It is commonly defined as a body mass index (BMI) of ≥30 kg/m^2, but other indexes such as waist circumference and waist to hip ratio have been used. It is an established risk factor for cardiovascular disease, and it has been associated with dyslipidemia and abnormalities in lipoprotein metabolism. However, it is not yet established how obesity affects postprandial lipid levels.

Obesity is associated with insulin resistance, favoring catabolism and lipolysis [16]. Hence, it may be expected that obesity is associated with postprandial lipemia. In our previous unpublished study, we have found that there was no significant difference in postprandial lipid response in obese subjects compared to normal-weight subjects. Interestingly, postprandial lipid levels were actually slightly lower in the obese group compared to the normal group. This study used BMI to classify obese subjects, and different results were seen in studies that focused on abdominal obesity. Abdominal obesity has been known to be a risk factor for cardiovascular disease [17], and it has been demonstrated that abdominal obesity is associated with prolonged and amplified postprandial lipid levels [18]. Interestingly, postprandial lipemia can be seen in abdominal obesity despite normal fasting levels of TG [18, 19].

5. Role of postprandial lipemia in endothelial inflammation and dysfunction

Postprandial lipemia is hypothesized to be a risk factor for cardiovascular disease by inducing endothelial dysfunction [20]. The vascular endothelial lining functions to maintain adequate blood flow and regulate coagulation and inflammation. Endothelial dysfunction signifies any disturbance to the vasodilatory response of the endothelium and impairment of its antithrombotic and antiproliferative function [21]. This eventually translates to atherosclerosis and CVD. Several studies have shown that intake of high-fat meals can induce an increase in postprandial TG levels and impair endothelial function [22, 23].

Postprandial lipemia promotes atherogenesis and endothelial dysfunction by contributing to the inflammatory state in the endothelial environment [24]. Postprandial lipemia has also been shown in in vitro and in vivo studies to activate leukocytes promoting adherence to endothelial walls and migration to the subendothelial space, therefore promoting atherosclerosis. VLDL, IDL, and chylomicron remnants have been shown to cause endothelial inflammation and promote increase in pro-inflammatory cells within the vascular walls. TG and TGRLs also induce pro-inflammatory cytokines that induce vascular cell adhesion molecule (VCAM)-1 expression in endothelial cells and monocyte adhesion. Lipolysis of TGRLs by the enzyme lipoprotein lipase (LPL) along with the endothelium produces by-products that are pro-inflammatory and pro-atherogenic. Lipolysis produces oxidized free fatty acids that promote endothelial inflammation, vascular apoptosis, and reactive oxygen species (ROS). Inflammation in the endothelium increases permeability and uptake of VDL in the vascular wall [25].

Maggi et al. have shown that postprandial levels of remnant lipoproteins (RLP) and TG contribute to endothelial dysfunction as measured by flow-mediated dilatation (FMD) of the brachial artery. They have demonstrated that the increase in postprandial RLP and TG levels was associated to the decrease in FMD. In addition, the peak level of RLP at 6 hours after meal coincided with the maximal endothelial dysfunction [26]. Their findings are supported by similar

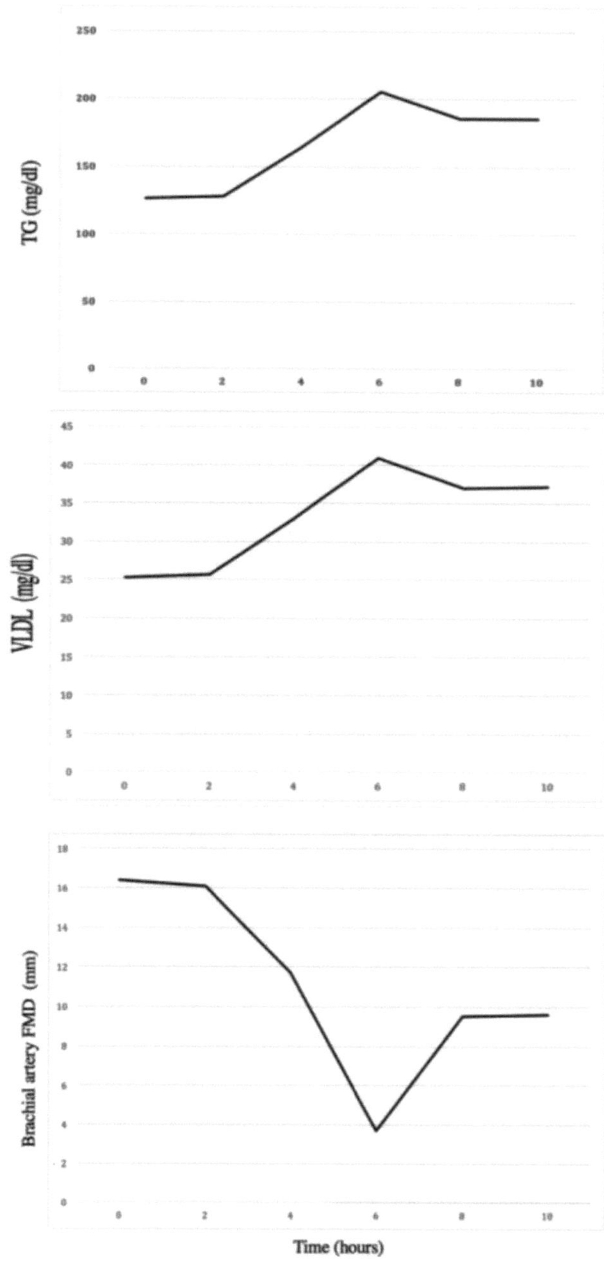

Figure 2.
The result from a study by Caringal et al. showing trends of lipid levels and brachial artery flow-mediated dilatation (FMD) after a standard diet.

results in a study by Caringal et al. that investigated the relationship between postprandial lipid levels and endothelial dysfunction using FMD as surrogate marker. Five high-risk subjects with normal fasting lipid levels were given a standard low-fat diet. Interestingly, it was observed that even though the fasting lipid levels were normal, the peaking of TG and VLDL 6 hours postprandially and the decrease in HDL postprandially appear to coincide with the decrease in brachial artery FMD [27] (**Figure 2**).

A study by Giannattasio et al. involving 16 asymptomatic hypertriglyceridemic and 7 normotriglyceridemic controls showed attenuation of arterial vasodilatory response following a high-fat meal among subjects with dyslipidemia. This reflects postprandial impairment of endothelial function after a high-fat meal [23].

6. Postprandial lipemia and CV events

Lipid-lowering therapy focusing on LDL-C reduction has been proven to reduce coronary events and stroke [28]. However, with the evidences of association of postprandial lipemia, specifically TG and RLP with endothelial dysfunction, it is important to assess their role in morbidity and mortality.

In a prospective cohort by Nordertgaard et al., involving a large number of white women and men of Danish descent, they have found that elevated levels of nonfasting triglyceride were associated with increased risk for CV events. They have specifically demonstrated that increasing levels of nonfasting TG were associated with progressively increasing hazard ratio for myocardial infarction (MI), ischemic heart disease (IHD), and death. In addition, they have also demonstrated that remnant lipoprotein cholesterol increases as nonfasting TG increase [29]. A study by Bansal et al. further supports the role of TG in predicting CV events. They have demonstrated that both fasting and nonfasting TG are risks for CV events. However, because HDL-C level is a confounding variable, after adjusting to HDL-C, they have seen that compared to fasting TG, nonfasting TG has a stronger independent relationship with cardiovascular events. Interestingly, they also demonstrated in secondary analyses that TG levels 2–4 hours postprandially had the strongest association with CV events [30]. This can be explained by the possibility that peaking of endothelial dysfunction coincides with peaking of postprandial lipemia [26]. Also, most studies mentioned have noted that peaking of postprandial TG and RLPs occurred 4 hours after a meal [5, 6, 26, 27]. On the contrary, in a study by Kats et al. involving 559 participants who underwent oral fat challenge, they have found that none of the measures of postprandial change were associated with incident CVD events. However, the study is inadequately powered [31]. Hence, there is a need for more robust prospective studies to clearly demonstrate the role and extent of postprandial lipemia effect on CV events. At present, the evidences should be enough to effect change in the way me manage dyslipidemia.

7. Treatment

Optimal treatment goals for postprandial lipid levels that will result to risk reduction have not been determined. At present, most guidelines are focused on LDL-C reduction and use fasting lipid profile. LDL-C target goals also depend on risk stratification, with extremely high-risk patients recommended to decrease LDL-C to as low as 55 mg/dl and low-risk patients to <130 mg/dl [32].

Normal TG levels have been set to be <150 mg/dl during the fasting state [32]. In a study by White et al. that aimed to determine optimal nonfasting TG levels involving middle-aged and older apparently healthy women, the diagnostic threshold for nonfasting hypertriglyceridemia is seen to be at 175 mg/dL [33].

8. Diet

The importance of lifestyle modification cannot be overemphasized. Patients with dyslipidemia are advised to have reduced-calorie diet. Saturated and trans fats should also be minimized [32]. In addition, it has been found that a minimum of 10 hours is needed for postprandial lipids to return to fasting or baseline levels [5]. Hence, to avoid prolonged exposure to elevated levels of postprandial lipids, fatty meals should be avoided or should at least be spaced 12 hours accordingly.

9. Statins

Statins are considered one of the first-line treatments for dyslipidemia. It has been established that statins are efficacious in lowering fasting lipids and that statin treatment has resulted to significant reductions in cardiovascular morbidity and mortality. Some studies also have proven that statins can be used to lower postprandial lipid levels. However, in our study, we found that even on low fat diet, statin treatment, and normal fasting lipids, triglyceride and VLDL peaking and plateauing were still observed in patients with cardiovascular disease [34]. Furthermore, Schaefer et al. did a comparative study among statins and their efficacy in lowering postprandial levels. They have found that atorvastatin was significantly more effective in lowering LDL cholesterol and non-high-density lipoprotein cholesterol than all other statins and significantly more effective than all statins, except for simvastatin, in lowering triglyceride and remnant lipoprotein cholesterol. At 40 mg/day, atorvastatin was significantly more effective than all statins, except for lovastatin and simvastatin, in lowering cholesterol levels in small LDL, and was significantly more effective than all statins, except for simvastatin, in increasing cholesterol in large HDL and in lowering LDL particle numbers [35].

10. Fibrates

In a study by Cavallero et al., it has been found that fenofibrate normalized the abnormal postprandial response and improved the fasting lipoprotein abnormalities in patients with type 2 diabetes [36]. This is supported by the study of Ooi et al., which showed that fibrate treatment resulted to a significant decrease in remnant lipoprotein levels postprandially [37].

11. Orlistat

A study by Turker et al. involving normolipidemic, obese women with normal glucose tolerance suggests that 12 weeks of treatment with orlistat 120 mg/d plus low-calorie diet was associated with a 4.1-fold change from baseline in PPL [38]. Abejuela et al. have shown that orlistat abolishes the peaking of TC, TG, and HDL after a 50% OFCT [6]. In a study by Gabriel et al. which compared the effects of orlistat on the postprandial lipid levels after sequential high-fat meals in healthy individuals with normal fasting lipid levels, they have seen that administration of orlistat abolished the significantly sustained postprandial rise of TG and VLDL levels in healthy individuals who were fed sequential 50% fat meals. Specifically, they have seen that in the control group, there is a significant postprandial rise in the levels of TG and VLDL beginning at 4 hours after breakfast that was sustained until 9 hours for TG and up to 10 hours for VLDL postprandially. In contrast, only one significant rise in both TG and VLDL levels was noted in the group given orlistat [5].

12. Ezetimibe

Ezetimibe is usually given to statin-intolerant patients or used in combination with statin to lower cholesterol, primarily LDL. There are evidences that it can also improve postprandial lipemia. In a study by Bozetto et al., they have shown that ezetimibe when given with simvastatin produces greater decrease in LDL cholesterol compared to simvastatin alone and produces a significant decrease in chylomicron lipid content both at fasting and postprandially, a significant decrease in chylomicron postprandial apoB-48, and significant fasting and postprandial decreases in the cholesterol content of VLDL, IDL, and LDL [39]. Yunoki et al. have demonstrated that a 4-week treatment with ezetimibe suppressed the postprandial peaking of TG, remnant lipoprotein, and apoB-48. Furthermore, they have shown that FMD reduction, which signifies endothelial dysfunction, also decreased with treatment [40].

13. Conclusion

We recognize that postprandial dyslipidemia is an undertreated disorder. Although robust prospective clinical trials are lacking, there is still increasing evidence of the clinical significance of postprandial dyslipidemia as a risk factor for CV disease. Clearly, postprandial elevations of lipids, specifically TG and TRLs, result to endothelial dysfunction and atherosclerosis. These result to increase in morbidity and possible mortality due to cardiovascular diseases. This should translate to a paradigm shift in the diagnosis and treatment of dyslipidemia. Presently, statins, fibrates, ezetimibe, and orlistat in sequential or combination regimen or as needed (orlistat) are possible treatment options for postprandial dyslipidemia in addition to proper diet and exercise. However, studies that focus on treatment of postprandial lipemia with measurement of solid clinical outcomes such as cardiovascular events and mortality should be undertaken. **Table 1** summarizes our recommendation.

Recommendations	
Diagnosis	• In addition to fasting lipid profile, postprandial lipid profile should also be determined, especially for patients at risk for cardiovascular disease • In high-risk individuals such as those with diabetes mellitus and those with diagnosed cardiovascular disease, postprandial lipid profile should routinely be evaluated • Postprandial lipid profile should include total cholesterol, TG, and HDL
Target	• Postprandial values must approximate normal fasting levels
Treatment	• Fibrates are the first-line drug of choice for postprandial lipemia with hypertriglyceridemia • Elevated postprandial total cholesterol should be treated with high-intensity statin • Ezetimibe can be considered if inadequately controlled by fibrates and statins • Orlistat as needed may be taken prior to a fatty meal

Table 1.
Summary of recommendations on the diagnosis and management of postprandial lipemia.

Conflict of interests

The authors have no conflicts of interests.

Author details

Neil Francis Amba and Leilani B. Mercado-Asis*
Section of Endocrinology and Metabolism, Department of Medicine, Faculty of Medicine and Surgery, University of Santo Tomas, Manila, Philippines

*Address all correspondence to: lmasis@ust.edu.ph

References

[1] Dominiczak MH. Lipoprotein Metabolism and Atherogenesis. Medical Biochemistry Fouth ed. Saunders; 2014. pp. 214-234

[2] Katsuyuki N, Takamitsu N, Yoshiharu T, Takeaki N, et al. Post-prandial lipoprotein metabolism: VLDL vs chylomicrons. Clinica Chimica Acta. 2011;**412**:1306-1318

[3] Stanhope KL, Schwarz JM, Keim NL, et al. Consuming fructose-sweetened, not glucose sweetened, beverages increase visceral adiposity and lipids and decreases insulin sensitivity in overweight/obese humans. The Journal of Clinical Investigation. 2009;**119**:1322-1334

[4] So T, Mercado-Asis LB, Zacarias MB, et al. A comparison of dose response postprandial lipid profile of healthy filipino subjects after an oral fat challenge test of varying fat contents. Philippine Journal of Internal Medicine. 2004;**42**:1-7

[5] Gabriel FS, Samson C, Abejuela Z, Sicat-Gabriel PR, Sumpio JP, Zacarias MB, et al. Post prandial effect of orlistat on the peaking of lipid level after sequential high fat meals. International Journal of Endocrinology and Metabolism. 2012;**10**(2):458-463

[6] Abejuela ZR, Macaballug AG, Sumpio JP, Zacarias MB, Mercado-Asis LB. Orlistat abolishes postprandial lipid peaking. International Journal of Endocrinology and Metabolism. 2009;**3**:179-186

[7] Rosenson RS, Helenowski IB, Tangney CC. Heterogeneous post prandial lipoprotein responses in the metabolic syndrome, and response to fenofibrate therapy. Cardiovascular Drugs and Therapy. 2010;**24**:439-447

[8] Cohn J, McNamara J, Cohn S, Ordovas J, Schaefer E. Postprandial plasma lipoprotein changes in human subjects of different ages. Journal of Lipid Research. 1988;**29**:469-479

[9] Lopez-Mirandal J, Williams C, Lairon D. Dietary, physiological, genetic and pathological influences on postprandial lipid metabolism. British Journal of Nutrition. 2007;**98**:458-473

[10] Shukla A. Postprandial lipid abnormalities in type 2 diabetes mellitus, a study at NGMC, Kohalpur. Journal of Nepalgunj Medical College. 2015;**13**:21-24

[11] Arca M. Alterations of intestinal lipoprotein metabolism in diabetes mellitus and metabolic syndrome. Atherosclerosis Supplements. 2015;**17**:12-16

[12] Castro-Caringal J, Mendoza E, Mercado-Asis LB. Correlation of postprandial lipemia with postprandial hyperglycemia and poor glycemic control among patients with type 2 diabetes mellitus. Philippine Journal of Internal Medicine. 2015;**53**(4):1-4

[13] Nakamura A, Monma Y, Kajitani S, Noda K, Nakajima S, Endo H, et al. Effect of glycemic state on postprandial hyperlipidemia and hyperinsulinemia with coronary artery disease. Heart and Vessels. 2016;**31**(9):1446-1455

[14] Asiam M, Aggarwal S, Sharnma KK, Galay V, Madhu SV. Postprandial hypertriglyceridemia predicts development of insulin resistance, glucose in tolerance and type 2 DM. PLoS One. 2016;**11**(1):e0145730

[15] Rivellese A, De Natale C, Di Lucrezia M, Lidia P, Ciro L, Sylvana C, et al. Exogenous and endogenous postprandial lipid

abnormalities in type 2 diabetic patients with optimal blood glucose control and optimal fasting triglyceride levels. The Journal of Clinical Endocrinology & Metabolism. 2004;**89**(5):2153-2159

[16] Singla P, Bardoloi A, Parkash A. Metabolic effects of obesity: A review. World Journal of Diabetes. 2010;**1**(3):76-88

[17] Frayn K. Insulin resistance, impaired postprandial lipid metabolism and abdominal obesity a deadely triad. Medical Principles and Practice. 2002;**11**(suppl 2):31-40

[18] Mekki N, Christofilis MA, Charbonnier M, Atlan-Gepner C, Defoort C, Juhel C, et al. Influence of obesity and body fat distribution on postprandial lipemia and triglyceride-rich lipoprotein in adult women. The Journal of Clinical Endocrinology and Metabolism. 1999;**84**:184-191

[19] Watts GF, Chan DCF, Barrett PHR, Martins IJ, Redgrave TG. Preliminary experience with a new stable isotope breath test for chylomicron remnant metabolism: A study in central obesity. Clinical Science. 2001;**101**:683-690

[20] Matsumoto S, Gotoh N, Hishinuma S, Abe Y, Shimizu Y, Katano Y, et al. The role of hypertriglyceridemia in the development of atherosclerosis and endotheliasl dysfunction. Nutrients. 2014;**6**:1236-1250

[21] Murray T, Yang E, Brunner G, Kumar A, Lakkis N, Misra A, et al. Post prandial effects on arterial stiffness parameters in healthy young adults. Vascular Medicine. 2015;**20**(6):501-508

[22] Blendea M, Bard M, Sowers J, Winer N. High-fat meal impairs vascular compliance in a subgroup of young healthy subjects. Metabolism Clinical and Experimental. 2005;**54**:1337-1344

[23] Giannattasio C, Zoppo A, Gentile G, Failla M, Capra A, Maggi M, et al. Acute effect of high-fat meal on endothelial dysfunction in moderately dislipidemic subjects. Arteriosclerosis, Thrombosis, and Vascular Biology. 2005;**25**:406-410

[24] Burdge G, Clader P. Plasma cytokine response during the postprandial period: A potential causal process in vascular disease? British Journal of Nutrition. 2005;**93**:3-9

[25] Lacroix S, Des RC, Tardif J, Nigam A. The role of oxidative stress in postprandial dysfunction. Nutrition Research Reviews. 2012;**25**:288-301

[26] Maggi FM, Raselli S, Grigore L, Redaelli L, Fantappiè S, Catapano AL. Lipoprotein remnants and endothelial dysfunction in the postprandial phase. The Journal of Clinical Endocrinology and Metabolism. 2004;**89**(6):2946-2950

[27] Castro-Caringal JA, Valera L, Llave K, Samson C, Ramirez M, Zacarias M, Mercado-Asis LB. Flow-mediated dilatation of brachial artery is inversely correlated with the postprandial peaking of triglyceride and very low-density lipoprotein. Unpubished

[28] Baigent C, Keech A, Kearney PM, Blackwell L, Buck G, Pollicino C, et al. Efficacy and safety of cholesterol-lowering treatment: Prospective meta-analysis of date from 90,056 participants in 14 randomised trials of statins. Lancet. 2005;**366**(9493):1267-1278. Epub 2005 Sept 27

[29] Nordertgaard B, Benn M, Schnohr P, Tybjaerg-Hansen A. Nonfasting triglycerides and risk of myocardial infarction, ischemic heart disease, and death in men and women. JAMA. 2007;**298**(3):299-308

[30] Bansal S, Buring JE, Rifai N, Mora S, Sacks FM, Ridker PM. Fasting

compared with non-fasting triglycerides and risk of cardiovascular events in women. JAMA. 2007;**298**:309-316

[31] Kats D, Sharrett A, Ginsberg H, Nambi V, Ballantyne C, Hoogeveen R, et al. Postprandial lipemia and the risk of coronary heart disease and stroke: The Atherosclerosis Risk in Communities (ARIC) Study. BMJ Open Diabetes Research and Care. 2017;**5**:e000335

[32] Jellinger P, Handelsman Y, Rosenblit P, Bloomgarden Z, Fonseca V, Garber A, et al. American association of clinical endocrinologists and American college of endocrinologist guidelines for management of dyslipidemia and prevention of cardiovascular disease. CPG for managing dyslipidemia and prevention of CVD. Endocrine Practice. 2017;**23**(Suppl 2)

[33] White K, Moorthy M, Akinkuolie A, Demier O, Ridker P, Cook N, et al. Identifying an optimal cutpoint value for the diagnosis of hypertriglyceridemia in the nonfasting state. Clinical Chemistry. 2015;**61**(9):1156-1163

[34] Samson CE, Galia AL, Llave KI, Zacarias, MB, Mercado-Asis LB. Postprandial peaking and plateauing of triglycerides and VLDL in patients with underlying cardiovascular diseases despite treatment. International Journal of Endocrinology and Metabolism. 2012;**10**:587-593

[35] Schaefer EJ, McNamara JR, Tayler T, Daly JA, Gleason JL, Senman LJ, et al. Comparisons of effects of statins (atorvastatin, fluvastatin, lovastatin, pravastatin, and simvastatin) on fasting and postprandial lipoproteins in patients with coronary heart disease versus control subjects. The American Journal of Cardiology. 2004;**93**(1):31-39

[36] Cavallero E, Dachet C, Assadolahi F, Martin C, Navarro N, Ansquer JC, et al. Micronized fenofibrate normalizes the enhanced lipidemic response to a fat load in patients with Type 2 DM and optimal glucose control. Atherosclerosis. 2003;**166**:151

[37] Ooi TC, Cousins M, Ooi DS, Nakajima K, Edwards AL. Effect of fibrates on postprandial remnant-like particles in patients with combined hyperlipidemia. Atherosclerosis. 2004;**172**:375

[38] Turker I, Demirag NG, Tanaci N, Tutar N, Kirbas I. Effects of orlistat plus diet on postprandial lipemia and brachial artery reactivity in normolipidemic, obese women with normal glucose tolerance: A prospective, randomized, controlled study. Current Therapeutic Research, Clinical and Experimental. 2006;**67**(3):159-173

[39] Bozetto G, Annuzzi A, Della Corte G, Patti L, Cipriano B, Mangione A, et al. Ezetimibe beneficially influences fasting and postprandial triglyceride-rich lipoproteins in type 2 diabetes. Atherosclerosis. 2011;**217**(1):142-148

[40] Yunoki K, Nakamura N, Miyoshi T, Enko K, Kohno K, Morita H, et al. Ezetimibe improves postprandial hyperlipemia and its induced endothelial dysfunction. Atherosclerosis. 2011;**217**(2):486-491

Section 3

Special Topics in the Management of Dyslipidemia

Chapter 6

Alternative Natural Management of Dyslipidemia

Abdullah Glil Alkushi

Abstract

In hypercholesterolemic patients, besides therapeutic treatments, alternative treatments can be used such as lifestyle changes, e.g. avoiding smoking, regular exercise, and consuming a diet rich in fiber and low in trans saturated and saturated fats. There are also certain plant products, such as the gum residue guggulipid, that are used in India as a traditional medicine to reduce blood cholesterol levels. Similarly, red yeast rice and rice bran oil have been observed to reduce elevated cholesterol levels. Other herbal products have also been investigated for their role in lowering cholesterol levels, as well as various other herbs and spices such as ginger and turmeric. Another herbal remedy available for reducing high cholesterol levels is the leaf extract of *Cynara scolymus*, commonly known as artichoke thistle. *Cynara cardunculus* var. *scolymus*, or globe artichoke, is mainly cultivated as a food crop. It has an important effect on reducing plasma cholesterol and low-density lipoprotein levels.

Keywords: alternative medicine, lifestyle changes, natural plants, Chinese medicine, vitamins and minerals

1. Dyslipidemia and Lifestyle

Hypercholesterolemia (HC) is defined as the increase in the levels of cholesterol in the blood. As per the recommendation of the expert panel of the National Cholesterol Education Program, desirable blood cholesterol levels should be <200 mg/dL. Levels ranging between 200 and 239 mg/dL are considered as borderline for cholesterol levels, and individuals with blood cholesterol levels above 240 mg/dL are considered hypercholesterolemic [1]. HC occurs due to both environmental and genetic factors [2]. According to familial HC, environmental factors mainly include obesity and diets rich in saturated fats, whereas genetic factors comprise the additive effects of several genes or defects in a single gene [3–5]. Elevated cholesterol levels in the blood not only cause coronary heart disease but can also lead to stroke and damage to the brain [6, 7]. High cholesterol has also been linked to peripheral vascular disease, in which fat is deposited mainly in the arteries that lead to the legs and feet [8]. HC is also linked to type 2 diabetes and hypertension [9, 10].

In hypercholesterolemic patients, besides therapeutic treatments, alternative treatments can be used such as lifestyle changes, e.g. avoiding smoking, regular exercise, and consuming a diet high in fiber and low in trans saturated and saturated fats. Similarly, red yeast rice and rice bran oil have been observed to reduce elevated cholesterol levels. Other herbal products have also been investigated for their role in lowering cholesterol levels, as well as various other herbs and spices such as ginger and turmeric.

Another herbal remedy is the leaf extract of *Cynara scolymus*, commonly known as artichoke thistle. *Cynara cardunculus* var. *scolymus*, or globe artichoke, is mainly cultivated as a food crop. It has important effects in reducing plasma cholesterol and low-density lipoprotein (LDL) levels. Also, many vitamins and minerals help to reduce and control fat and cholesterol levels.

These will be discussed in this chapter.

1.1 Lifestyle changes

One of the most important things in the natural treatments of dyslipidemia is to reduce body weight and take regular exercise [11], which will help to regulate blood cholesterol [12] and decrease the high risk of developing cardiovascular diseases, especially coronary heart disease [13].

1.2 Stopping smoking

This is important in controlling high blood cholesterol, decreasing the risk of coronary heart disease, and improving high-density lipoprotein (HDL) cholesterol [14]. The mechanism of cigarette smoking will have an effect on lipid profile and enhance oxidation of plasma LDL, which leads to endothelial function impairment.

1.3 Alcohol intake

Alcohol has adverse effects on cholesterol and lipid levels, including raising serum triglyceride and HDL cholesterol levels. It has a minimum effect on LDL cholesterol but has effects on the body, including hepatic toxicity, cardiomyopathy, impaired reflexes, and psychosocial problems [15].

1.4 Exercise

Exercise is important in reducing the chance of developing heart disease. It is also important to reduce body weight, which can lead to reduced levels of fat and cholesterol [11].

Physical activity and exercise can be an important factor to improve cholesterol levels, increase HDL, and reduce LDL and triglycerides [16].

Aerobic exercise can generally improve lipid profile [17].

Moderate intensity aerobic exercise and an increase in physical activity in healthy people for more than 30 minutes for 5 days a week are important to maintain low LDL, cholesterol, and triglyceride levels, as well as increase HDL levels [18, 19].

In dyslipidemia especially in older or disabled individuals, increasing physical activity for more than 30 minutes for 5 days a week, moderate-intensity aerobic exercise [19], and high-intensity resistance exercises can all reduce LDL and triglycerides and increase HDL [20].

The beneficial effects of regular physical activity and exercise on cholesterol levels are important in the management of dyslipidemia and can lead to reducing the risks of heart attacks, strokes, and coronary heart disease.

2. Food that should be avoided

1. Food containing too much sugar and carbohydrates, which stimulate the liver to produce more cholesterol, should be avoided.

2. Hydrogenated and trans fats increase cholesterol and the risk of cardiovascular diseases.

3. Red meat and animal products increase the risk of dyslipidemia.

3. Food and dyslipidemia

Foods that help to decrease dyslipidemia are shown in **Tables 1** and **2**.

3.1 Dietary fiber intake

Dietary fiber (DF) intake provides many health benefits. However, the average fiber intake for US children and adults is less than half of the recommended levels. Individuals with high intakes of DF appear to be at significantly lower risk for developing coronary heart disease, stroke, hypertension, diabetes, obesity, and certain gastrointestinal diseases. Increasing fiber intake lowers blood pressure and serum cholesterol levels.

The effect of dietary soluble fiber on serum cholesterol levels has been extensively documented and promoted. The main mechanisms for the cholesterol-lowering effects of water-soluble and -insoluble DFs include binding and excretion of bile acids (BAs) in the small intestine. The cholesterol-reducing effect of water-insoluble DF, such as lignin or citric fiber, is rather low compared to water-soluble DF and is mainly based on direct binding of BAs. In the small intestine the BAs are bound to the insoluble DF and excreted from the enterohepatic circulation together with the undigested DF, which results in a lowering of blood cholesterol levels.

In addition, soluble fibers are known to bind to BAs in the small intestine, thereby removing them from the body and reducing the rate of BA recycling. The loss of BAs in the stool stimulates the liver to increase cholesterol uptake from the circulation to replenish the BA supply. As a result, concentrations of serum total and LDL cholesterol are reduced, while HDL cholesterol and triglycerides are generally unaffected [21].

3.2 Omega-3

Omega-3 fatty acids are presented in two formulas:

- Docosahexaenoic acid (DHA)

- Eicosapentaenoic acid (EPA)

Omega-3 fatty acids are important in reducing triglycerides and non-HDL cholesterol [22–24].

Reducing triglycerides and cholesterol helps to reduce atherosclerosis [25–28].

Using omega-3 fatty acids has benefits in metabolic abnormality associated with non-alcoholic fatty liver in patients with hyperlipidemia [29].

3.3 Garlic

Garlic (*Allium sativum*) belongs to onion genes. It used as an herb medication for various diseases. It has major roles in decreasing risk factors of cardiovascular diseases like high blood pressure and high serum lipids [30–33].

Plant name	Type	Effects on lipid profile
Dietary fiber	Food	Lowers LDL and cholesterol levels
Omega-3	Food	Lowers cholesterol and triglyceride levels
Garlic	Food	Lowers cholesterol and triglyceride levels
Red yeast rice	Food	Lowers cholesterol level
Chinese medicine	Herbal	Lowers hyperlipidemia
Artichoke	Food	Lowers cholesterol level
Fenugreek	Herbal	Lowers cholesterol level
Gum residue guggulipid	Herbal	Lowers LDL and cholesterol levels
Ginger	Food	Lowers cholesterol level

Table 1.
Foods and herbals and their effects on lipid profiles.

Name	Type	Effects on lipid profile
Vitamin B3 (niacin)	Water-soluble vitamin	Lowers LDL, cholesterol, and triglyceride levels
Vitamin B5	Water-soluble vitamin	Lowers LDL, cholesterol, and triglyceride levels
Vitamin C	Water-soluble vitamin	Protects against LDL oxidation
Vitamin D	Fat-soluble vitamin	Reduces the risk of arterial blockage
Magnesium	Mineral	Protects against LDL oxidation
Manganese	Mineral	Protects against LDL oxidation
Zinc	Mineral	Protects against dangerous lipoproteins and promotes HDL
Selenium	Mineral	Protects against dangerous lipoproteins
Copper	Mineral	Protects against dangerous lipoproteins
Coenzyme Q10	Mineral	Protects against dangerous lipoproteins
Chromium	Mineral	Increases HDL level
Choline	Mineral	Controls HDL level
Inositol	Mineral	Lowers LDL and triglyceride levels
Lipoic acid	Mineral	Lowers LDL and protects against cholesterol oxidation
Carnitine	Mineral	Lowers LDL and triglyceride levels

Table 2.
Vitamins and minerals and their effects on lipid profiles.

Garlic reduces cholesterol, LDL, and triglyceride levels by inhibiting cholesterol biosynthesis in the liver and LDL oxidation [34–38].

There are a few side effects associated with using garlic such as allergic dermatitis [39] and its interference with oral anticoagulant drugs [39].

3.4 Read yeast rice

Red yeast rice is a product of rice and is found in China and many Asian countries where it is used as a traditional medicine [40, 41].

Biochemically it contains polyketides, unsaturated fatty acids, phytosterols, pigments, and monacolins [41, 42]. It lowers cholesterol by inhibiting 5-hydroxy-3-methylglutaryl-coenzyme A (HMG-CoA) reductase, which is the rate-limiting step for cholesterol synthesis in the liver. This component, especially monacolins, is chemically similar to lovastatin (a drug used to treat hypercholesteremia) [41, 43].

3.5 Chinese medicine

Traditional Chinese medicine (TCM) has been used in clinical practice for many centuries. Chinese medicine has shown good effects for human health and treating many diseases. Recently, TCM has shown a beneficial effect for treating dyslipidemia; however, its mechanism remains unclear or totally unknown. Many studies on dyslipidemia with a single Chinese herb showed that TCM can improve phlegm, dampness, and blood stasis syndromes in patients with hyperlipidemia, therefore it has a beneficial effect for lowering hyperlipidemia monomers or effective extracts [44–46].

One study [46] showed that Chinese herbs, which have effects on hyperlipidemia, have four beneficial characteristics:

1. Clearing heat and removing toxicity, for example, Radix et Rhizoma Rhei, Rhizoma Polygoni Cuspidati, Semen Cassia, Coptis chinensis, Scutellaria baicalensis, Gynostemma pentaphyllum, and Radix Puerariae.

2. Promoting blood circulation and removing blood stasis, for example, Fructus crataegi, red yeast rice, Rhizoma, Radix *Salvia miltiorrhizae*, and Turmerone.

3. Eliminating dampness and phlegm, for example, Rhizoma Alismatis, plantain seed, and folium nelumbinis.

4. Increasing body energy, for example, Radix Astragali, Radix Ginseng, and Radix polygoni multiflori.

3.6 Artichoke

Another herbal remedy available for reducing high cholesterol levels is the leaf extract of *Cynara scolymus*, commonly known as artichoke thistle. *Cynara cardunculus* var. *scolymus*, or globe artichoke, is mainly cultivated as a food crop. It is a perennial plant that is largely native to the Mediterranean region in Southern Europe and Northern Africa, and the Canary Islands. In addition to food, artichoke is used in tea and liqueur preparation. Studies on the medicinal properties of artichoke have been continuing over the last six decades. Several in vitro and in vivo studies have investigated the effect of artichoke leaf extract (ALE), especially cymarine, in reducing plasma cholesterol levels [47–50]. Along with cymarine, the antiatherosclerotic effect of luteolin-rich artichoke extract reduces LDL oxidation in a dose-dependent manner [51]. A dose-dependent inhibition of cholesterol biosynthesis, using ALE, was also shown in primary-cultured rat hepatocytes [52].

In addition to in vitro and in vivo studies, randomized controlled studies have assessed the effects of the oral administration of ALE in hypercholesterolemic patients. Bundy et al. assessed the effect of ALE on plasma lipid levels and general well-being in healthy individuals with mild to moderate HC [53]. The participants of the study received 1280 mg of ALE daily (four tablets of 320 mg) for 12 weeks. The majority of participants were females, and almost 90% of them were more than 40 years old. The plasma cholesterol levels were found to be reduced by 4.2%

in the group administered ALE, whereas they increased by 1.9% in the placebo group. No significant difference in LDL cholesterol, HDL cholesterol, or triglycerides was observed between the groups. Englisch et al. conducted a similar study among 18–70-year-old hypercholesterolemic patients [54]. In addition to treatment with cholesterol-reducing drugs, participants were prohibited from antibiotic treatment. The intervention group received 1800 mg of ALE for 6 weeks. Total cholesterol levels were reduced by 18.5% in the group administered with ALE as compared to a 8.6% reduction in the placebo group. In addition to atherosclerosis, HC can affect organs such as kidneys. Studies in rats have shown that cholesterol can increase the incidence of glomerulosclerosis, and in vitro cell culture studies using human glomerular cells revealed the possible mechanisms that are involved in lipid-influenced glomerular damage [55]. Another study showed that treating HC in obese rats reduced their glomerular injuries [56]. Similar observations have also been made in studies with humans. Individuals with high triglycerides or a lecithin–cholesterol acyltransferase deficiency gradually developed renal failure due to glomerulosclerosis [57].

C. cardunculus leaf extract (CCL) not only has cholesterol-reducing capacity but also reduces blood glucose levels and repairs impaired kidney function and damage. These findings are significant particularly because HC results in further complications such as diabetes and kidney damage, both of which can be treated effectively with artichoke [50].

The hypercholesterolemic properties of artichoke involve inhibition of the enzyme HMG-CoA reductase. By lowering blood cholesterol levels and improving lipid profile, experts believe that artichoke can reduce the risks of arteriosclerosis and coronary heart disease and found that both CCL and *C. cardunculus* pulp extract.

decrease the concentration of the respective enzymes (an increase in levels of aspartate transaminase (AST), alanine aminotransferase (ALT), and alkaline phosphatase (ALP) are indicators of liver dysfunction), hence serving hepatoprotective and regenerating effects [58]. Thus, it was concluded that artichoke has a beneficial effect on cardiovascular and liver disease.

3.7 Fenugreek seeds

Fenugreek (*Trigonella foenumgraecum*) has an effect on cholesterol and blood sugar. It is a good source of dietary fiber and has beneficial effects on decreasing cholesterol levels in blood and the liver [59, 60].

The mechanism of the lipid-lowering effect of fenugreek seeds is due to the presence of 4-hydroxyisoleucine, a branched chain amino acid [61], and its action on adipocytes and liver cells, which leads to decreased triglycerides, cholesterol, and LDL [62, 63].

3.8 Gum residue guggulipid

A gum resin of the tree *Commiphora mukul*, used for the management of obesity and lipid disorders, is centuries old [64]. The extract of this gum resin, designated guggulipid, has lipid-lowering effects in normal and hyperlipidemic animals (rats, rabbits, and monkeys) [65, 66].

In humans, many studies of the effect of gum resin gumsome in response to guggul treatment were observed in of patients in India [67].

In the United States, studies showed that 18% of patients showed a response to guggulipid treatment, with a decrease in LDL levels of more than 5% [68].

Variations in the results of clinical studies are due to many factors such as ethnic and genetic backgrounds, dietary restraints, and lifestyle [69].

3.9 Ginger

Ginger (*Zingiber officinale*) is a traditional natural plant, which has many characteristics such as decreasing lipid levels, antiplatelet aggregation, and antioxidant and anticarcinogenic qualities [70]. Several studies show that ginger can lower high cholesterol levels in animals. In humans a few study results showed the effects of using ginger in patients with high cholesterol and in the treatment of dyslipidemia [71].

4. Vitamins and minerals

4.1 Vitamin B3 (niacin)

Niacin is a water-soluble vitamin. It effectively lowers the atherogenic lipoprotein(a) by decreasing the rate of synthesis in the liver and lowering the level of cholesterols as well as triglycerides [72, 73]. It is important in reducing the incidence of cardiovascular disease.

4.2 Vitamin B5

Vitamin B5 is a water-soluble vitamin, which is also called pantothenic acid. It is important in the synthesis of coenzyme A, as well as lowering LDL metabolism and reducing triglycerides [74, 75].

4.3 Vitamin C

Vitamin C is a water-soluble vitamin and is essential for repairing tissues and enzyme production. It has a role in lipid metabolism, protects LDL from oxidation, and lowers atherosclerosis and lipoprotein(a) in some people [76, 77].

4.4 Vitamin D

Vitamin D is a fat-soluble vitamin and has an important function in the body, including calcium homeostasis and suppressing foam cell formation, which reduces the risk of arterial blockage [78, 79] therefore reducing cardiovascular disease problems.

4.5 Magnesium

Magnesium protects LDL from being oxidized [80, 81].

4.6 Manganese

Manganese is a cofactor to the antioxidant superoxide dismutase that repairs damage to blood vessels caused by oxidized LDL [82, 83].

4.7 Zinc

Zinc protects against dangerous lipoproteins that lead to vascular inflammation and plaque formation. It also controls the gene that makes HDL [84, 85].

4.8 Selenium

Selenium prevents postprandial change in lipoproteins, which makes them easy to oxidize and become harmful [86, 87].

4.9 Copper

Many copper-dependent enzymes affect lipoprotein metabolism that build up fats and cholesterol in arteries [88–90].

4.10 Coenzyme Q10

Coenzyme Q10 lowers lipoprotein(a) and improves dyslipidemia medicine [91, 92].

4.11 Chromium

Chromium increases HDL levels and cooperates with niacin (B3) for dyslipidemia [93–95].

4.12 Choline

Choline controls HDL metabolism due to the enzyme lecithin cholesterol acyltransferase that has beneficial effects on lipoprotein metabolism [96, 97].

4.13 Inositol

Inositol lowers LDL levels, especially in patients with metabolic syndrome. It also lowers triglyceride levels [98–100].

4.14 Lipoic acid

Lipoic acid lowers LDL levels and protects against oxidized cholesterol [101, 102].

4.15 Carnitine

Carnitine lowers triglycerides, LDL, and the atherogenic lipoprotein(a) by transporting fatty acids into cells so that they can be used as energy [103–105].

5. Conclusion

Besides pharmacological treatments for HC, using alternative treatments may help to increase the effectiveness of drugs. Alternative treatments can help to alter sedentary lifestyles and include exercise, stopping smoking, and eating a number of foods (omega-3, garlic, red yeast rice), herbs (Chinese medicine), vitamins (B, B5, C, and D), and many minerals.

Author details

Abdullah Glil Alkushi
Department of Anatomy, Faculty of Medicine, Umm Al-Qura University, Makkah, Saudi Arabia

*Address all correspondence to: dr.alkushi@gmail.com

References

[1] Goodman DS, Hulley SB, Clark LT, et al. expert panel on detection, evaluation, and treatment of high blood cholesterol in adults. The expert panel. Archives of Internal Medicine. 1988;**148**:36-69

[2] Bhatnagar D, Soran H, Durrington PN. Hypercholesterolaemia and its management. BMJ. 2008;**337**:a993

[3] Innerarity TL, Mahley RW, Weisgraber KH, Bersot TP, Krauss RM, Vega GL, et al. Familial defective apolipoprotein B-100: A mutation of apolipoprotein B that causes hypercholesterolemia. Journal of Lipid Research. 1990;**31**:1337-1349

[4] Grundy SM. George Lyman Duff Memorial Lecture. Multifactorial etiology of hypercholesterolemia. Implications for prevention of coronary heart disease. Arteriosclerosis and Thrombosis. 1991;**11**:1619-1635

[5] Sniderman AD, Tsimikas S, Fazio S. The severe hypercholesterolemia phenotype: Clinical diagnosis, management, and emerging therapies. Journal of the American College of Cardiology. 2014;**63**:1935-1947

[6] Clark LT. Cholesterol and heart disease: Current concepts in pathogenesis and treatment. Journal of the National Medical Association. 1986;**78**:743-751

[7] Navi BB, Segal AZ. The role of cholesterol and statins in stroke. Current Cardiology Reports. 2009;**11**:4-11

[8] Cooke JP. The pathophysiology of peripheral arterial disease: Rational targets for drug intervention. Vascular Medicine. 1997;**2**:227-230

[9] Kwiterovich PO. Primary and secondary disorders of lipid metabolism in pediatrics. Pediatric Endocrinology Reviews. 2008;**5**(Suppl 2):727-738

[10] Ivanovic B, Tadic M. Hypercholesterolemia and hypertension: Two sides of the same coin. American Journal of Cardiovascular Drugs. 2015;**15**:403-414

[11] National Cholesterol Education Program. Second Report of the Expert Panel on Detection, Evaluation, and Treatment of High Blood Cholesterol in Adults (Adult Treatment Panel II). Bethesda, Md: National Cholesterol Education Program, National Institutes of Health, National Heart, Lung, and Blood Institute; 1993. DHSS Publication No. (NIH) 93-3095:5

[12] Yeshurun D, Gotto AM Jr. Hyperlipidemia: Perspectives in diagnosis and treatment. Southern Medical Journal. 1995;**88**:379-391

[13] The lipid research clinics coronary primary prevention trial results. I. Reduction in incidence of coronary heart disease. Lipid Research Clinics Program. JAMA. 1984;**251**:351-364

[14] Adam D, Gepner M, Megan E. Effect of smoking and smoking cessation on lipid and lipoprotein: Outcomes from a randomized clinical trial. American Heart Journal. 2011;**161**(1):145-151

[15] Ahmed SM, Clasen ME, Donnelly JF. Management of dyslipidemia in adults. American Family Physician. 1998;**57**(9):2192-2204

[16] Ferguson MA, Alderson NL, Trost SG, et al. Effects of four different single exercise sessions on lipids, lipoproteins, and lipoprotein lipase. Journal of Applied Physiology. 1998;**85**(3):1169-1174

[17] Kraus W, Houmard J, Duscha B, et al. Effects of the amount and intensity

of exercise on plasma lipoproteins. The New England Journal of Medicine. 2002;**347**(19):1483-1492

[18] Aadahl M, Kjaer M, Jørgensen T. Associations between overall physical activity level and cardiovascular risk factors in an adult population. European Journal of Epidemiology. 2007;**22**(6):369-378

[19] Fett C, Fett W, Marchini J. Circuit weight training vs jogging in metabolic risk factors of overweight/obese women. Arquivos Brasileiros de Cardiologia. 2009;**93**(5):519-525

[20] Lira F, Yamashita A, Uchida M, et al. Low and moderate, rather than high intensity strength exercise induces benefit regarding plasma lipid profile. Diabetology and Metabolic Syndrome. 2010;**2**:31

[21] Osfor MMH, Ashsh AM, ElSawy NA, Qusty NFH, Alkushi AG. Effect of wheat bran consumption on serum lipid profile of hypercholesterolemia patients residence in Holly Makah. Asian Journal of Natural & Applied Sciences. 2016;**5**(1):1-9

[22] Harris WS, Ginsberg HN, Arunakul N, et al. Safety and efficacy of Omacor in severe hypertriglyceridemia. Journal of Cardiovascular Risk. 1997;**4**(5-6):385-391

[23] Pownall HJ, Brauchi D, Kilinc C, et al. Correlation of serum triglyceride and its reduction by omega-3 fatty acids with lipid transfer activity and the neutral lipid compositions of high-density and low-density lipoproteins. Atherosclerosis. 1999;**143**(2):285-297

[24] Maki KC, Orloff DG, Nicholls SJ, et al. A highly bioavailable omega-3 free fatty acid formulation improves the cardiovascular risk profile in high-risk, statin-treated patients with residual hypertriglyceridemia (the ESPRIT trial). Clinical Therapeutics. 2013;**35**(9):1400-1411

[25] Jorgensen AB, Frikke-Schmidt R, Nordestgaard BG, et al. Lossof-function mutations in APOC3 and risk of ischemic vascular disease. The New England Journal of Medicine. 2014;**371**(1):32-41

[26] TG and HDL Working Group of the Exome. Sequencing Project NHLaBI. Loss-of-function mutations in APOC3, triglycerides, and coronary disease. The New England Journal of Medicine. 2014;**371**(1):22-31

[27] Khetarpal SA, Rader DJ. Triglyceride-rich lipoproteins and coronary artery disease risk: New insights from human genetics. Arteriosclerosis, Thrombosis, and Vascular Biology. 2015;**35**(2):e3-e9

[28] Dewey FE, Gusarova V, O'Dushlaine C, et al. Inactivating variants in ANGPTL4 and risk of coronary artery disease. The New England Journal of Medicine. 2016;**374**(12):1123-1133

[29] Qin Y, Zhou Y, Chen S-H, et al. Fish oil supplements lower serum lipids and glucose in correlation with a reduction in plasma fibroblast growth factor 21 and prostaglandin E2 in nonalcoholic fatty liver disease associated with hyperlipidemia: A randomized clinical trial. PLoS One. 2015;**10**(7):e0133496. DOI: 10.1371/journal.pone.0133496. Herder C, editor

[30] Ackermann RT, Mulrow CD, Ramirez G. Garlic shows promise for improving some cardiovascular risk factors. Archives of Internal Medicine. 2001;**161**(6):813

[31] Qidwai W, Ashfaq T. Role of garlic usage in cardiovascular disease prevention: An evidence-based approach. Evidence-Based Complementary and Alternative Medicine. 2013;**2013**:1-9. Article ID 125649

[32] Khoo YSK, Aziz Z. Garlic supplementation and serum cholesterol:

A meta-analysis. Journal of Clinical Pharmacy and Therapeutics. 2009;**34**(2):133-145

[33] Osamor PE, Owumi BE. Complementary and alternative medicine in the management of hypertension in an urban Nigerian community. BMC Complementary and Alternative Medicine. 2010;**10**(1):36

[34] Zhang XH, Lowe D, Giles P. A randomized trial of the effects of garlic oil upon coronary heart disease risk factors in trained male runners. Blood Coagulation & Fibrinolysis. 2001;**12**(1):67-74

[35] Lau BHS. Suppression of LDL oxidation by garlic compounds is a possible mechanism of cardiovascular health benefit. The Journal of Nutrition. 2006;**136**(3):765-768

[36] Duda G, Suliburska J, Pupek-Musialik D. Effects of short-term garlic supplementation on lipid metabolism and antioxidant status in hypertensive adults. Pharmacological Reports. 2008;**60**(2):163

[37] Zeng T, Zhang CL, Zhao XL. The roles of garlic on the lipid parameters: A systematic review of the literature. Critical Reviews in Food Science and Nutrition. 2013;**53**(3):215-230

[38] Jahan F, Nanjib K, Qidwai W. Role of garlic in dyslipidemia: An evidence based review. Scientific Journal of Biological Sciences. 2015;**4**(5):36-42

[39] Steiner M, Khan AH, Holbert D, Lin RI. A double-blind crossover study in moderately hypercholesterolaemic men that compared the effect of aged garlic extract and placebo administration on blood lipids. The American Journal of Clinical Nutrition. 1996;**64**:866-870

[40] Burke FM. Red yeast rice for the treatment of dyslipidemia. Current Atherosclerosis Reports. 2015;**17**(4):495

[41] Francini-Pesenti F et al. Red yeast rice in the long-term treatment of hypercholesterolemia. A single-center experience. Acta Scientific Agriculture. 2017;**1**(3):16-18

[42] Patel S. Functional food red yeast rice (RYR) for metabolic syndrome amelioration: A review on pros and cons. World Journal of Microbiology and Biotechnology. 2016;**32**(5):2035-2042

[43] Zhang Z et al. Cytotoxic monacolins from red yeast rice, a Chinese medicine and food. Food Chemistry. 2016;**202**:262-268

[44] Shi HX, Li QH. Research progress of traditional Chinese medicine treatment of hyperlipidemia. Journal of Medical Forum. 2007;**28**(10):123-124

[45] Jiang JG. The clinical study progress of Chinese herbal medicine for hyperlipidemia. Journal of Practical Traditional Chinese Medicine. 2008;**24**(9):614-615

[46] Guo M, Liu Y, Gao ZY, Shi DZ. Chinese herbal medicine on dyslipidemia: Progress and perspective. Evidence-based Complementary and Alternative Medicine. 2014;**2014**:1-11

[47] Wojcicki J, Winter S. Effect of preparation Cynarex on the blood serum lipids level of the workers exposed to the chronic action of carbon disulphide. Medycyna Pracy. 1975;**26**:213-217

[48] Wójcicki J. Effect of 1,5-dicaffeylquinic acid (cynarine) on cholesterol levels in serum and liver of acute ethanol-treated rats. Drug and Alcohol Dependence. 1978;**3**:143-145

[49] Wojcicki J, Samochowiec L, Kosmider K. Influence of an extract from artichoke (*Cynara scolymus* L.) on the level of lipids in serum of aged men. Herba Polonica. 1981;**27**:265-268

[50] Alkushi AG. Biological effect of Cynara cardunculus on kidney status of hypercholesterolemic rats. Pharmacognosy Magazine. 2017;**13**:S430-S436

[51] Brown JE, Rice-Evans CA. Luteolin-rich artichoke extract protects low density lipoprotein from oxidation in vitro. Free Radical Research. 1998;**29**:247-255

[52] Gebhardt R. Inhibition of cholesterol biosynthesis in primary cultured rat hepatocytes by artichoke (*Cynara scolymus* L.) extracts. The Journal of Pharmacology and Experimental Therapeutics. 1998;**286**:1122-1128

[53] Bundy R, Walker AF, Middleton RW, Wallis C, Simpson HC. Artichoke leaf extract (Cynara scolymus) reduces plasma cholesterol in otherwise healthy hypercholesterolemic adults: A randomized, double blind placebo controlled trial. Phytomedicine. 2008;**15**:668-675

[54] Englisch W, Beckers C, Unkauf M, Ruepp M, Zinserling V. Efficacy of artichoke dry extract in patients with hyperlipoproteinemia. Arzneimittel-Forschung. 2000;**50**:260-265

[55] Gröne EF, Walli AK, Gröne HJ, Miller B, Seidel D. The role of lipids in nephrosclerosis and glomerulosclerosis. Atherosclerosis. 1994;**107**:1-13

[56] Kasiske BL, O'Donnell MP, Cleary MP, Keane WF. Treatment of hyperlipidemia reduces glomerular injury in obese Zucker rats. Kidney International. 1988;**33**:667-672

[57] Samuelsson O, Mulec H, Knight-Gibson C, Attman PO, Kron B, Larsson R, et al. Lipoprotein abnormalities are associated with increased rate of progression of human chronic renal insufficiency. Nephrology, Dialysis, Transplantation. 1997;**12**:1908-1915

[58] Header EA, ElSawy NA, Alkushi AG. Biological effect of Cynara cardunculus on liver and heart status for hypercholesterolemic rats. Australian Journal of Basic and Applied Sciences. 2017;**11**(2):41-49

[59] Nadkarni KM. Trigonella foenum graecum: Indian materia. Médica. 1993;**1240**:1249

[60] Kumar K, Kumar S, Datta A, Bandyopadhyay A. Effect of fenugreek seeds on glycemia and dyslipidemia in patients with type 2 diabetes mellitus. International Journal of Medical Science and Public Health. 2015;**4**(7):997-1000

[61] Belaid Nouira Y, Bakhta H, Bouaziz M. Study on the lipid profile and the parieto-temporal lipid peroxidation in $AlCl_3$ mediated neurotoxicity: the modulatory effect of the fenugreek seeds. Lipids in Health and Disease. 2012;**11**:6

[62] Jetle L, Harvey L, Eugeni K, Leven SN. The 4-hydroxy isoleucine plant-derived treatment for metabolic syndrome. Current opinion treatment for the metabolic syndrome. Current Opinion in Investigational Drugs. 2000;**10**:353-358

[63] Sharma MS, Choudhary PR. Hypolipidemic effect of fenugreek seeds and its comparison with atorvastatin on experimentally induced hyperlipidemia. Journal of the College of Physicians and Surgeons–Pakistan. 2014;**24**(8):539-542

[64] Dev S. Ethnotherapeutics and modern drug development. The potential of Ayurveda. Current Science. 1997;**73**:909-928

[65] Satyavati GV. Gum guggul (Commiphora mukul)—The success story of an ancient insight leading to a modern discovery. The Indian Journal of Medical Research. 1988;**87**:327-335

[66] Singh K, Chander R, Kapoor NK. Stimulation of low density lipoprotein receptor activity in liver membrane of guggulsterone treated rats. Pharmacological Research. 1990;**22**:37-44

[67] Deng R. Therapeutic effects of guggul and its constituent guggulsterone: Cardiovascular benefits. Cardiovascular Drug Reviews. 2007;**25**:375-390

[68] Szapary PO, Wolfe ML, Bloedon LT, et al. Gugulipid for the treatment of hypercholesterolemia: A randomized controlled trial. Journal of the American Medical Association. 2003;**290**:765-772

[69] Ramachandran C, Nair SM, Quirrin K-W, Melnick SJ. Hypolipidemic effects of a proprietary Commiphora Mukul gum resin extract and medium-chain triglyceride preparation (GU-MCT810). Journal of Evidence-Based Complementary & Alternative Medicine. 2013;**18**(4):248-256

[70] Ellen RL, McPherson R. Long-term efficacy and safety of fenofibrate and a statin in the treatment of combined hyperlipidemia. The American Journal of Cardiology. 1998;**81**:60-65

[71] Fuhrman B, Rosenblat M, Hayek T, Coleman R, Aviram M. Ginger extract consumption reduces plasma cholesterol, inhibits LDL oxidation and attenuates development of atherosclerosis in atherosclerotic, apolipoprotein E-deficient mice. The Journal of Nutrition. 2000;**130**:1124-1131

[72] Seed M, O'Connor B, Perombelon N, et al. The effects of nicotinic acid and acipimox on lipoprotein (a) concentration and turnover. Atherosclerosis. 1993;**101**:61-68

[73] Kostner K, Gupta S. Niacin: A lipid polypill? Expert Opinion on Pharmacotherapy. 2008;**9**:2911-2920

[74] McRae M. Treatment of hyperlipoproteinemia with pantethine: A review and analysis of efficacy and tolerability. Nutrition Research. 2005;**25**:319-333

[75] Rumberger J, Napolitano J, Azmumano I, et al. Pantethine, a derivative of vitamin B(5) used as a nutritional supplement, favorably alters low-density lipoprotein cholesterol metabolism in low- to moderate-cardiovascular risk North American subjects: A triple-blinded placebo and diet-controlled investigation. Nutrition Research. 2011;**31**:608-615

[76] Woollard K, Loryman C, Meredith E, et al. Effects of oral vitamin C on monocyte: Endothelial cell adhesion in healthy subjects. Biochemical and Biophysical Research Communications. 2002;**294**:1161-1168

[77] Shariat S, Mostafavi S, Khakpour F. Antioxidant effects of vitamins C and E on the low density lipoprotein oxidation mediated by myeloperoxidase. Iranian Biomedical Journal. 2013;**17**:22-28

[78] Riek A, Oh J, Bernal-Mizrachi C. Vitamin D regulates macrophage cholesterol metabolism in diabetes. The Journal of Steroid Biochemistry and Molecular Biology. 2010;**121**:430-433

[79] Guasch A, Bulló M, Rabassa A, et al. Plasma vitamin D and parathormone are associated with obesity and atherogenic dyslipidemia: A cross-sectional study. Cardiovascular Diabetology. 2012;**11**:149

[80] Sherer Y, Bitzur R, Cohen H, et al. Mechanisms of action of anti-atherogenic effect of magnesium: Lessons from a mouse model. Magnesium Research. 2001;**14**:173-179

[81] Maier J. Low magnesium and atherosclerosis: An evidence-based link. Molecular Aspects of Medicine. 2003;**24**:137-146

[82] Takabe W, Li R, Ai L, et al. Oxidized low-density lipoprotein-activated c-Jun NH2-terminal kinase regulates manganese superoxide dismutase ubiquitination: Implication for mitochondrial redox status and apoptosis. Arteriosclerosis, Thrombosis, and Vascular Biology. 2010;**30**:436-441

[83] Perrotta I, Perrotta E, Sesti S, Cassese M and Mazzulla S, et al. MnSOD expression in human atherosclerotic plaques: An immunohistochemical and ultrastructural study. Cardiovascular Pathology. 2013;**22**:428-437. Epub ahead of print

[84] Wu J, Wu Y, Reaves S, et al. Apolipoprotein A-I gene expression is regulated by cellular zinc status in hep G2 cells. The American Journal of Physiology. 1999;**277**:C537-C544

[85] Shen H, MacDonald R, Bruemmer D, et al. Zinc deficiency alters lipid metabolism in LDL receptor deficient mice treated with rosiglitazone. The Journal of Nutrition. 2007;**137**:2339-2345

[86] Natella F, Fidale M, Tubaro F, et al. Selenium supplementation prevents the increase in atherogenic electronegative LDL (LDL minus) in the postprandial phase. Nutrition, Metabolism, and Cardiovascular Diseases. 2007;**17**:649-656

[87] Kaur H, Bansal M. Studies on scavenger receptors under experimental hypercholesterolemia: Modulation on selenium supplementation. Biological Trace Element Research. 2011;**143**:310-319

[88] Hamilton I, Gilmore W, Strain J. Marginal copper deficiency and atherosclerosis. Biological Trace Element Research. 2000;**78**:179-189

[89] Wildman R, Mao S. Tissue-specific alteration in lipoprotein lipase activity in copper-deficient rats. Biological Trace Element Research. 2001;**80**:221-229

[90] DiSilverstro R, Joesph E, Zhang W, et al. A randomized trial of copper supplementation effects on blood copper enzyme activities and parameters related to cardiovascular health. Metabolism. 2012;**61**: 1242-1246

[91] Langsjoen P, Langsjoen A. The clinical use of HMG CoA reductase inhibitors and the associated depletion of coenzyme Q10. A review of animal and human publications. BioFactors. 2003;**18**:101-111

[92] Cicero A, Derosa G, Miconi A, et al. Possible role of ubiquinone in the treatment of massive hypertriglyceridemia resistant to PUFA and fibrates. Biomedicine & Pharmacotherapy. 2005;**59**:312-317

[93] Press R, Geller J, Evans G. The effect of chromium picolinate on serum cholesterol apolipoprotein fractions in human subjects. The Western Journal of Medicine. 1990;**152**:41-45

[94] Sealls W, Penque B, Elmendorf J. Evidence that chromium modulates cellular cholesterol homeostasis and ABCA1 functionality impaired by hyperinsulinemia—Brief report. Arteriosclerosis, Thrombosis, and Vascular Biology. 2011;**31**:1139-1140

[95] Sundaram B, Singhal K, Sandhir R. Anti-atherogenic effect of chromium picolinate in streptozotocin-induced experimental diabetes. Journal of Diabetes. 2013;**5**:43-50

[96] Vance D. Role of phosphatidylcholine biosynthesis in the regulation of lipoprotein homeostasis. Current Opinion in Lipidology. 2008;**19**:229-234

[97] Kunnen S, Van Eck M. Lecithin:cholesterol acyltransferase:

Old friend or foe in atherosclerosis? Journal of Lipid Research. 2012;**53**:1783-1799

[98] Jariwalla R. Inositol hexaphosphate (IP6) as an anti-neoplastic and lipid-lowering agent. Anticancer Research. 1999;**19**:3699-3702

[99] Maeba R, Hara H, Ishikawa H, et al. Myo-inositol treatment increases serum plasmalogens and decreases small dense LDL, particularly in hyperlipidemic subjects with metabolic syndrome. Journal of Nutritional Science and Vitaminology. 2008;**54**:196-202

[100] Minozzi M, Nordio M, Pajalich R. The combined therapy myo-inositol plus D-chiro-inositol, in a physiological ratio, reduces the cardiovascular risk by improving the lipid profile in PCOS patients. European Review for Medical and Pharmacological Sciences. 2013;**17**:537-540

[101] Zhang Y, Han P, Wu N, He B, Lu Y, Li S, et al. Amelioration of lipid abnormalities by α-lipoic acid through antioxidative and anti-inflammatory effects. Obesity (Silver Spring). 2011;**19**(8):1647-1653

[102] Harding S, Rideout T, Jones P. Evidence for using alpha-lipoic acid in reducing lipoprotein and inflammatory related atherosclerotic risk. Journal of Dietary Supplements. 2012;**9**:116-127

[103] Sirtori C, Calabresi L, Ferrara S, et al. L-carnitine reduces plasma lipoprotein(a) levels in patients with hyper Lp(a). Nutrition, Metabolism, and Cardiovascular Diseases. 2000;**10**:247-251

[104] Derosa G, Cicero AF, Gaddi A, Mugellini A, Ciccarelli L, Fogari R. The effect of L-carnitine on plasma lipoprotein(a) levels in hypercholesterolemic patients with type 2 diabetes mellitus. Clinical Therapeutics. 2003; **25**(5):1429-1439

[105] Malaguarnera M, Vacante M, Avitabile T, et al. L-Carnitine supplementation reduces oxidized LDL cholesterol in patients with diabetes. The American Journal of Clinical Nutrition. 2009;**89**:71-76

Chapter 7

The Role of Niacin in the Management of Dyslipidemia

Joseph M. Keenan

Abstract

Niacin or nicotinic acid has been used for the management of dyslipidemia for over 50 years, and it is the first medication that has been shown to reduce both coronary disease events and mortality. It is unique among the various lipid therapies in that it can not only reduce all of atherogenic lipid fractions (total cholesterol, low-density lipoprotein, very low-density lipoprotein, non-HDL lipoproteins, and triglycerides), but is also the most effective agent for raising high-density lipoprotein (specifically Apolipoprotein A-1). It is also the only lipid therapy that can lower lipoprotein (a). Niacin also has non-lipid benefits that improve vascular health and reduce atherogenesis. Niacin therapy was initially hampered by a high incidence of side effects, especially flushing, but this has largely been overcome by extended-release formulations and dosing and administering properly. Despite the failure of two recent clinical trials to show benefit of combining niacin with statins, there are many trials that support using niacin as monotherapy or in combination with other lipid agents including statins. Niacin is also the cheapest lipid agent available, and with the epidemic of cardiovascular disease in the world, it offers great value in the population-wide management of this health problem.

Keywords: niacin, nicotinic acid, HDL-C, Lp(a), niacin formulations

1. Background: early niacin trials

Niacin or vitamin B3 comes in two forms, nicotinamide and nicotinic acid (NA), but only NA has lipid management benefits. The recommended daily allowance of vitamin B3 for nutritional benefit is only 20–30 mg/day, but the dose needed for lipid benefits is much higher and depends on whether one is using immediate-release (IRNA) 3000–6000 mg/day or extended-release (ERNA) 1000–2000 mg/day formulations [1, 2]. The lipid benefits of NA were discovered serendipitously in the 1940–1950s when mega-doses of vitamins were being used in the management of mental health disorders. It was noted that high doses of NA lowered total cholesterol significantly. It was at that same time that elevated cholesterol was found to be associated with increased risk of cardiovascular disease (CVD) that led to the early trials of NA for management of dyslipidemia. Investigators in those early studies did not know what the mechanism of action of NA was but they were impressed that not only did NA lower total cholesterol by 20+%, but also specifically lowered beta lipoprotein cholesterol (LDL-C), raised alpha lipoprotein cholesterol (HDL-C), and lowered triglycerides (TG) [3, 4].

IntechOpen

It became evident at that time that high cholesterol was not only associated with increased risk of CVD, but also diet and lifestyle interventions were usually not adequate to reduce cholesterol levels. This led to a large clinical trial, The Coronary Drug Project, that was a head to head trial of the cholesterol lowering agents available then (Thyroxine, Estrogen-two forms, Clofibrate and IRNA). The study was conducted from 1969 to 1975 and had five treatment arms and a large placebo arm totaling 8341 subjects [5]. The thyroxine and both estrogen treatment arms were terminated early due to lack of benefit and the clofibrate arm had some lipid improvements that failed to show reduction in coronary events. The IRNA arm not only demonstrated significant improvements in clinically important lipid fractions (total cholesterol, LDL-C, HDL-C, and TG) but, more importantly, it had a significant decrease in coronary events compared to placebo group. In addition, long-term (15 years) follow-up showed 11% decrease in mortality in the IRNA group compared to the placebo [6]. The only negative aspect of the Coronary Drug Project was the high incidence of flushing (>60%) in the IRNA treatment group. The immediate-release formulation of NA was used in that study, and, even though the majority of subjects were able to develop some level of tolerance, 8% had to drop out due to flushing.

2. NA mechanism of action

Nicotinic acid offers multiple clinical benefits to the lipid profile but the most unique and important is its ability to raise HDL-C. The 2017 Guidelines on the Management of Dyslipidemia list low HDL-C and a major risk factor for coronary disease because of important role of HDL-C in reverse cholesterol transport [7]. No agent is more potent at raising HDL-C than NA. NA not only NA raises HDL-C but also selectively prevents liver catabolism of apolipoprotein A-1, which is the key HDL lipoprotein needed for reverse cholesterol transport [8]. Thus NA increases both the capacity and the efficiency of HDL-C cholesterol transport. The liver is the site of synthesis of TG, very low-density lipoprotein (VLDL), lipoprotein (a) (Lp(a)), and LDL-C, and NA attaches to and antagonizes the hydroxycarboxylic acid-2 receptor of hepatocytes. This inhibits a hepatic microsomal enzyme (diacylglycerol acyltransferase-2) that is necessary for the final step in the production of those lipids [8]. Not only does NA reduce the beta lipoproteins that make up LDL-C,

Lipid benefits
-Lowers total cholesterol -Lowers LDL-C cholesterol (specifically low-density LDL-C) -Lowers triglycerides -Lowers Lp(a) -Raises HDL-C (specifically apolipoprotein A-1)
Non-lipid benefits
-Inhibits vascular inflammation/reduces reactive oxygen species -Reduces oxygenation of LDL-C -Reduces intravascular adhesion molecules and monocyte chemo-attractant protein-1 (atherogenesis initiators) -May reduce the size and functional recovery time of acute stroke
Ref. [7–9].

Table 1.
Summary of niacin lipid and non-lipid cardiovascular benefits.

but also more specifically NA reduces the small dense LDL-C particles that are most atherogenic. Furthermore, NA is one of the best agents to lower TG and is the only medication that significantly lowers Lp(a), which is also a significant independent risk factor for coronary disease [7].

In addition, in vitro research using human aortic endothelial cells has demonstrated impressive non-lipid benefits of NA in reducing risk of coronary disease. Researchers found that: (1) NA inhibits vascular inflammation by reducing reactive oxygen species, (2) NA reduces LDL-C oxidation making it less atherogenic, and (3) NA reduces vascular adhesion molecules and monocyte chemo-attractant protein-1, which decreases the attachment of monocytes and macrophages to the vascular wall, a key element in early atherogenesis [8]. An animal study demonstrated an additional non-lipid effect of NA, which is a neuroprotective benefit following stroke. The study involved inducing a stroke by middle cerebral artery occlusion in rats. Rats induced with NA within 2 hours of occlusion had a reduced volume of brain tissue damage and improved the functional recovery compared with controls [9] (**Table 1**).

3. Side effects of NA

Despite its many benefits, NA utilization can be hampered by a number of adverse side effects. The good news is virtually all NA side effects are reversible, and most can be minimized or eliminated by appropriate dosing and administration. The most common side effect is flushing and that is more common with IRNA and the initial doses of ERNA. Flushing is caused by release of prostaglandin D2 and prostaglandin E2 from Langerhans cells in the skin and macrophages [8]. In most persons, this flushing response can be minimized by proper dosing and administration (discussed later). William Parsons Jr., a co-investigator in the Coronary Drug Project and an early proponent of NA, was quite disappointed that many clinicians never learned "how to do" niacin resulting in higher dropout rates in NA therapy than that was warranted. This led him to writing a book, "Cholesterol Control Without a Diet! The Niacin Solution" for both lay and professional persons in an effort to educate all on proper NA administration [10].

Another side effect that is sometimes seen with ERNA therapy (but almost never with IRNA) is impaired liver function. This is due to methyl group depletion in the hepatocytes, secondary to the metabolic amidization in the liver of NA to nicotinamide [8]. This problem was shown to be preventable or reversible in most cases without loss of lipid benefit in studies using wax-matrix ERNA (WM-ERNA; Endur-Acin by Endurance Products Inc.) by either dose reduction or methyl group supplementation with methionine [11, 12]. Hepatic transaminase levels should be monitored during NA therapy. Modest transaminase level increases are acceptable, but NA dose reduction should be implemented if levels approach 2–3 times normal limits.

Increased blood glucose levels with NA therapy had raised concerns about its use in persons with diabetes or impaired glucose tolerance (metabolic syndrome). Blood glucose should be monitored in patients on NA treatment but that concern has been largely dismissed by the results from clinical trials. A controlled trial using WM-ERNA in non-diabetics showed only a 1% rise in baseline glucose levels at 6 weeks that returned to baseline by 6 months [13]. The AIM-HIGH trial that used polygel ERNA (PG-ERNA; Niaspan, AbbVie Inc.) specifically recruited persons with low HDL-C and high TG (metabolic syndrome or MS) found a 5% rise initially from baseline glucose levels that returned to baseline over 2 years, and there was no difference in the development of diabetes in the two treatment groups [14]. A post-hoc analysis of the Coronary Drug Project (that used IRNA) found that the subgroup of subjects with MS had comparable reduction in coronary events and long-term mortality to the other subjects in the IRNA treatment group [15]. The consensus is that the benefits of treating lipid risk factors in persons with MS or diabetes outweighs any modest increase that NA treatment may cause to insulin resistance.

There are a number of less common side effects with NA treatment most of which are manageable without discontinuing therapy. Gastrointestinal upset can occur in some individuals and may be due to increased acid production on NA treatment. This is usually managed by splitting the daily dose and taking it with meals. Acid blocking agents may also help. Hyperuricemia may also occur with NA treatment and uric acid levels should be monitored routinely along with blood glucose levels and liver function tests. Nicotinuric acid is a by-product of liver metabolism of NA and can complete with renal excretion of uric acid causing levels to rise. The clinician must decide whether the continued use of NA would require additional management of uric acid levels is worth the lipid benefits. Increased homocysteine levels can occur with NA treatment and these should also be monitored routinely during NA therapy. Hyper-homocysteinemia is also a risk factor for cardiovascular disease that can be managed by folic acid supplementation. Some persons may experience a rash with flushing that usually clears with the development of tolerance, and in a rare instance, a darkened patch of skin may occur (acanthosis nigricans). All of these side effects are completely resolvable/reversible by discontinuing NA if other management of the side effect is unsuccessful.

4. Selecting appropriate patients for NA therapy

As described above, the pleiotropic benefits of NA treatment make it an excellent choice for mixed dyslipidemias. One of the most prevalent forms of mixed dyslipidemia that is uniquely suited to NA treatment is MS (low HDL-C, high TG). A study of prevalence of MS in the United States showed 34% of all adults and 55% of persons over the age of 60 has MS [16]. An 8 year prospective study of cardiovascular risk (Framingham) in 3323 middle-aged adults in the United States found the risk of developing CVD over that 8 year period for persons with MS was 34% for men and 16% for women [17]. An epidemiology study of the prevalence of MS in European countries found it as high as 71.7% of adults in some countries and MS-associated CVD prevalence as high as 52% [18]. Thus, the prevalence and the high risk of CVD with MS make this a very large population of persons who would benefit from NA therapy, especially those persons with normal or modest elevations of LDL-C.

The problem of treating MS with NA as monotherapy is achieving the LDL-C goal for that person. Since cardiovascular risk assessment views MS as the equivalent of having a prior coronary event the LDL-C goal is usually more aggressive (e.g.70 mg/dl) and that can be difficult to achieve on NA alone. A meta-analysis in 2010 of NA studies using NA alone or in combination with other agents showed a 26% reduction in coronary events. In addition, they showed a decrease in coronary atherosclerosis in 92% of persons treated with NA, as well as a reduction in carotid intimal thickness of 17 mm per year of NA treatment [2]. Most of these studies were conducted prior to the introduction of statins for lipid management. The compliment of the lipid benefits of NA and the effective LDL-C lowering benefit of statin drugs led to clinical trials using PG-ERNA with statins which did demonstrate broad improvement of lipid profiles (decreased LDL-C, TG, Lp(a), and increased HDL-C) [19, 20]. Modeling of lipid therapy from these studies indicated that an ERNA with a statin would produce optimal lipid values for reducing coronary disease [21].

The early success in lipid profile improvement of combination trials of PG-ERNA/statin led to the development of two very large clinical trials of combination PG-ERNA/statin therapy that were intended to demonstrate conclusively the benefit of combined treatment on the reduction of cardiovascular events and mortality (Atherothrombosis Intervention in Metabolic Syndrome With Low HDL/High Triglycerides and Impact on Global Health Outcomes [AIM-HIGH] and Second Heart Protection Study—Treatment of HDL to Reduce the Incidence of Vascular Events [HPS-2 THRIVE]) [22, 23]. The much-anticipated results of those trials were very disappointing and not only failed to demonstrate reduction in vascular events but also appeared to show increased adverse events and side effects with that combination. Critics of these two trials pointed out major design flaws in both studies that raise serious questions about the validity of any conclusions drawn from study results. The AIM-HIGH trial was terminated early because of what was thought to be an increase in cerebrovascular accidents in the PG-ERNA/statin treatment group, which in later analysis was found to be an artifact [22]. The main conclusion of the AIM-HIGH trial was that the combined PG-ERNA/statin treatment group did not show a decrease in cardiovascular events. This, in fact, was not true for the subgroup who were in the highest tertile of baseline TG and the lowest tertile of baseline HDL-C, both lipid fractions that benefitted from the NA addition to treatment [24]. Another AIM-HIGH post-hoc analysis of remnant lipoproteins and HDL-C2 showed that the PG-ERNA/statin treatment group did demonstrate improvements that could confer benefit in prevention of cardiovascular events, but perhaps this was not able to be demonstrated because of early termination [25]. Others also point out that the Coronary Drug Project took 6 years to demonstrate a reduction in coronary events with NA therapy, so the failure of AIM-HIGH and HPS-2 THRIVE to demonstrate the same may have been due to early termination of these studies [26]. Also, one of the lipid benefits of adding NA to a statin is the additional lowering of LDL-C which did occur in the AIM-HIGH trial. However, this benefit was muted since the control group had a second LDL-C lowering drug (ezetimibe) added to their treatment to match any LDL-C lowering by NA in the treatment group [22].

The HPS-2 THRIVE trial was actually PG-ERNA in combination with Laropiprant, a prostaglandin DP1 receptor inhibitor that reduces the NA flushing side effect, and together this combination was added to statin therapy. The investigators had no idea when designing the study that the PG-ERNA/Laropiprant combination would cause such an increase in myopathies especially in Chinese subjects. Of the 25,673 study subjects over 11,000 were Chinese, and their annual incidence of myopathy was 800% greater than that European subjects on the same treatment [27]. Critics of the HPS-2 THRIVE trial felt the addition of Laropiprant to the NA treatment group confounded the outcomes and thus they do not accept it as a legitimate study of the combination of NA and statin therapy [26]. The main conclusion of the HPS-2 THRIVE study was similar to the AIM-HIGH study; that is, the addition of NA to statin therapy did not improve cardiovascular outcomes, and, in fact, resulted in an increase in serious adverse effects [23]. Despite the design flaws in these large trials, the consensus is that adding NA to statin therapy in persons who are already at their LDL-C goal does not improve clinical outcomes. These two large studies raised serious questions about what is the appropriate combination therapy with statins in persons who have not reached their LDL-C goal. While this controversy still lingers, many feel the effectiveness of NA in reducing LDL-C (especially small dense LDL-C particles) as well as the other lipid benefits as shown in earlier studies continues to make NA an appropriate combination with statins to achieve lipid goals and desired clinical endpoints [26].

Recent changes in recommendations of national cholesterol treatment guidelines in the United States have increased the number who are considered eligible to start statin therapy (absolute risk of cardiac event >7.5% over 10 years) to over 50 million persons [28]. The rate of statin intolerance (stopping therapy) in general population cholesterol intervention is 18–20% or about 10 million persons (statin intolerant) in the United States who are candidates for other lipid therapy interventions [29]. This represents another large target group that is appropriate for NA therapy since none of the other agents available have abroad range of lipid and non-lipid benefits for prevention of CVD [8, 26]. Some have suggested that proprotein-convertase subtilisin/kexin type 9 (PCSK-9) inhibitors be used when statin intolerance is encountered. At a cost of $15,000/year for PCSK-9 inhibitors and an estimated incremental cost of $330,000 per quality-adjusted life-years (QALYs), this option is very limited [30].

Perhaps the largest group of persons who would be logical candidates for NA lipid therapy globally are those whose risk scores indicate need to initiate lipid treatment but either they, individually, or their health system cannot afford statin treatment. Cardiovascular disease has grown at epidemic rates in developing countries and those countries account for over 80% of all cardiovascular deaths annually [31]. Using microsimulation modeling, analysts recently demonstrated that initiating statin therapy at the recommended 7.5% risk threshold would be an incremental cost-effectiveness ratio of $37,000 per QALYs gained [32]. This may be considered cost-effective in a developed country, but in a developing country this is prohibitive. Not only does NA have the broadest profile of lipid and non-lipid benefits for coronary disease/mortality reduction, it is also the cheapest available lipid lowering agent. Thus, it makes sense as a public health strategy for developing countries to initiate population level of lipid therapy intervention with NA monotherapy adding other agents as needed, and reserve initiation with statin therapy to the subset of persons with high/very high risk status.

Persons with isolated dyslipidemic fractions such as low HDL-C, or high TG are also reasonable candidates for NA therapy and NA is the only agent at present that can significantly lower Lp(a). A meta-analysis of clinical trials specifically targeting hypertriglyceridemia (two trials were NA monotherapy, one NA with fibrates) showed significant reduction in coronary events especially if high TG was associated with low HDL-C [33]. A meta-analysis of clinical trials of NA to lower Lp(a) showed significant reductions of 22–24%, and a case report of NA with a statin showed a dramatic 88% reduction [34, 35].

5. Choosing an NA formulation

The early clinical trials of NA used immediate-release formulations with good lipid results but many of those trials had unacceptably high drop-out rates due to flushing [36]. In an effort to reduce the flushing side effects, sustained-release NA formulations were developed. These did reduce flushing but continuous/sustained exposure of the liver to NA resulted in a high incidence of impaired liver function [36]. Researchers found that an intermediate (between immediate and sustained) or ERNA provided the best reduction in flushing side effects and also reduced the liver issues encountered with the more sustained-release formulations [36]. Another formulation that was made popular by its "no flush" claim is inositol hexanicotinate (six molecules of niacin attached to inositol). There are many NA products available on-line and over-the-counter that claim to be extended-release preparations but most of them have not been studied for safety, efficacy, and side effects in controlled clinical trials. Poon conducted an *in vitro* dissolution study of 19 non-prescription NA products comparing them to 1 prescription PG-ERNA product (Niaspan) [37]. He found wide variation in dissolution rates suggesting the *in vivo* NA release from these products would difficult to predict.

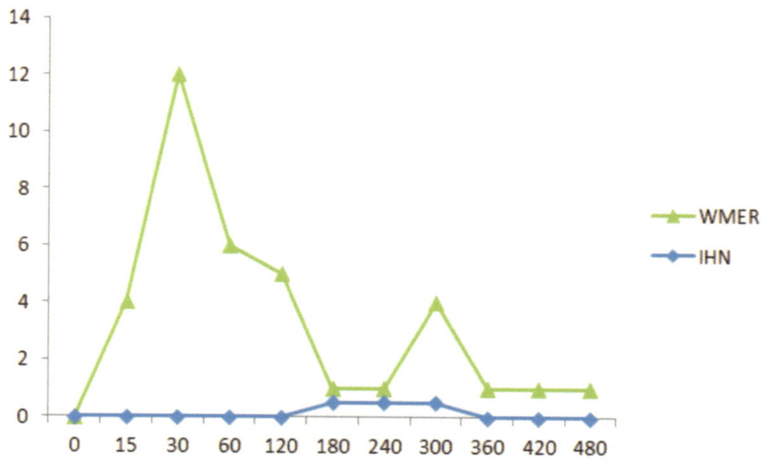

Figure 1.
Mean blood levels (ng/ml) over 8 hours of NA after single dose of 500 mg of wax-matrix nicotinic acid (WMER) and 500 mg dose of inositol hexanicotinate (IHN).

In selecting an NA product for clinical use, it is best to stay with products that have demonstrated safety and efficacy in clinical trials. The PG-ERNA, Niaspan, is the only NA formulation that has been approved by the US Food and Drug Administration for lipid therapy and is the standard by which other NA products are measured. It is by far the most extensively tested NA formulation having been used in both monotherapy and combined therapy with other agents including the AIM-HIGH and HPS-2 THRIVE studies. It has consistently demonstrated the desired lipid benefits and has typically had a total drop-out rate of 18–19% (9–10% due to flushing intolerance and 8–9% due to other adverse effects) [38]. Another polygel extended-release NA product, Slo-Niacin (Upsher-Smith Inc.) has also been extensively tested in clinical trials and was used in a large Veteran's Administration NA interchange study. Veterans who were on Niaspan (5321 subjects) were switched to Slo-Niacin and followed for 2 years. The results showed comparable safety/side effects and lipid benefits and Slo-Niacin had even greater lowering of TG [39]. A third NA product that uses a wax-matrix for its extended-release formulation is Endur-Acin (Endurance Products Inc). Endur-Acin has demonstrated comparable if not better lipid results compared the PG-ERNAs and it has exceptional safety and side effect rates with an average total drop-out rate of only 3–8% for 4 clinical trials totaling more than 400 subjects [11, 13, 40, 41]. Since age is one of the strongest non-lipid risk factors for CVD, it is worth noting that a post-hoc analysis of one of the Endur-Acin trials showed that older persons enjoyed even better lipid results than younger persons with no increase in side effects or drop-out rates [42]. The only clinical trial testing inositol NA as monotherapy showed its claim of "no flush" is a scam. In a head to head comparison trial with wax-matrix NA (Endur-Acin) that included pharmacokinetics of both agents, wax-matrix NA demonstrated an optimal extended-release and absorption curve over 8 hours and inositol NA had a flat line absorption curve demonstrating no bioavailability at all [41] (See **Figure 1**).

6. NA dosing and administration: "How to do" niacin

Guidelines recommend determining the patients risk score for likelihood of a coronary event in the next 10 years and discussing treatment options and goals before initiating treatment. Initiation of NA therapy also should be preceded by baseline check of lipids, blood glucose, hemoglobin A1C, uric acid, homocysteine, and liver transaminases to be sure the patient is an appropriate candidate. If you are primarily targeting low HDL-C with NA therapy, the most effective formulation is IRNA. Even though that form of NA has the highest rate of flushing it can be minimized in most persons by proper dosing and administration: (1) initiating therapy at a low dose (250–500 mg) and gradually increasing over 1–2 weeks to allow tolerance to develop, (2) giving aspirin with the dose of NA to block the prostaglandin response, and (3) giving the NA dose with meals to slow the rate of absorption. The Coronary Drug Project using IRNA had only an 8% drop-out rate due to flushing. Typically, IRNA dosing is advanced to at least 3000 mg/day for optimal HDL-C response but can be increased to as high as 6000 mg/day in divided doses with meals to reach goals as tolerated. Lipids and blood chemistries should be rechecked at 6 weeks and monitored at 6 week intervals until targeted dose has been reached. If chemistries remain within normal limits (liver transaminases acceptable up to three times, the upper limit of normal) then monitoring interval can be extended to 3 months once targeted dose has been reached. For most persons whose liver function tests approach/exceed three times the upper limit of normal, simply reduce dosage by half and recheck tests in 2 weeks. They are most likely sensitive to the amidization metabolism of NA in the liver and are becoming depleted of methyl groups. They will usually continue to have excellent lipid results at the lower dose and will also benefit from a diet rich in "methyl donor" foods (kale, berries, fish, nuts, etc.) or taking a methionine supplement. In the Endur-Acin versus inositol clinical trial six persons on Endur-Acin had dose reduction due to liver enzyme elevations, yet all had a good lipid response and five were able to reach their LDL-C goal [41]. If additional lipid lowering agents are needed, follow up can be adjusted to take into consideration monitoring that added agent or any possible interactions of agents.

For essentially all other NA lipid therapies (other than isolated low HDL-C), ERNA is better tolerated and more effective for the other lipid fractions. Initiating dosing for ERNA therapy is essentially the same as IRNA as listed above. Most of the PG-ERNA studies have used one time/day dosing at bedtime with a small snack for two reasons: (1) convenience (and it can be given at the time a statin is supposed to be given) and (2) to match the time of peak hepatic lipid synthesis. The PG-ERNAs (Niaspan and Slo-Niacin) also have a somewhat higher rate of flushing than the WM-ERNA (Endur-Acin) so giving it in a near fasting state may also reduce the chance of early breakdown of the polygel capsule that might happen with the increased peristaltic activity of a meal. Critics of the bedtime NA dosing used in the AIM-HIGH and HPS-2 THRIVE studies, however, point out that dosing NA in a fasting or near fasting state causes a drop in non-esterified fatty acids. This in turn can inadvertently cause a transient drop in blood glucose triggering release of epinephrine and hepatic gluconeogenesis which might have caused some of the negative results found in those studies [26]. Also, persons taking any ERNA should be cautioned to avoid consuming a hot beverage with dosing since that can accelerate NA release and risk flushing.

In targeting appropriate patients for NA lipid therapy, it is helpful to know what lipid changes to expect for typical dosing of NA. Increases in HDL-C are typically in the +12 to +22% range with an IRNA dose of 3000 mg or an ERNA (Niaspan, Slo-Niacin, Endur-Acin) dose of 1500–2000 mg with IRNA and Niaspan being toward the better response end. Decreases in LDL-C for those agents are typically in the −12 to −26% with Endur-Acin toward the better response end. Decreases in TG are typically −10 to −15% and Lp(a) about −18 to −22% [11, 43–45]. Knowing the patients baseline lipid/chemistry levels and their 10 year coronary risk score can help in choosing an NA agent and dosing strategy. A person with isolated low HDL-C would be a good candidate for IRNA or possibly Niaspan if they do not tolerate the flushing with IRNA. A person with MS, since they are considered higher risk for a coronary event (lower LDL-C goals), might do well to start on Endur-Acin and get the extra LDL-C benefit. In a clinical trial using Endur-Acin in persons with mild to moderate dyslipidemia 78% of persons with 0–1 cardiac risk factor and 44% of persons with 2 or more risk factors were able to get to their LDL-C goal along with the additional NA benefits in other lipid fractions [41]. A person whose baseline chemistries suggest glucose intolerance might best be placed on mealtime dosing to avoid reactive hypoglycemia and epinephrine release, and, of course, anyone with pre-existing liver function issues would best be started on IRNA. Management of side effects and adverse events from NA therapy are covered above (**side effects of NA**). Despite the bad press from the AIM-HIGH and HPS-2 THRIVE studies, NA has been used successfully with virtually every class of lipid lowering agent especially statins. With the possible exception of adding NA therapy to a person who is already at their LDL-C goal on statins, providers should feel comfortable adding other agents to NA or NA to other agents to achieve lipid goals [46, 47].

Last but not least in considering NA for lipid therapy is the cost. There are many very inexpensive NAs available in pharmacies, health supplement stores, and on-line, all claiming to lower cholesterol. But the patient should be advised to stay with those products that have been proven safe and effective in clinical trials, and specifically to avoid the NAs that claim "no flush" (inositol hexanicotinate) that have been proven "no benefit". Endur-Acin (WM-ERNA) and Slo-Niacin (PG-ERNA) are available on-line for only $8–9.00 USD/month for treatment (www.endur.com; www.slo-niacin.com). Niaspan is available only by prescription and is more expensive as are generic statins which are about 5–6 times more expensive. The cost may not be a big issue for persons with full drug coverage health insurance. But for others, even those with a co-pay, taking a medication that you will need for the rest of your life can be a substantial expense.

7. Conclusion

Nicotinic acid is the first dyslipidemia medication to reduce both CVD events and mortality. No other lipid medication has the breadth of lipid and non-lipid benefits for managing CVD risk. Specifically, NA is the best agent for raising HDL-C, one of the best agents for lowering TG and the only medication that can significantly lower Lp(a). This is in addition to ability of NA to significantly lower LDL-C, and non-HDL-C. Unique non-lipid benefits include reduction of LDL-C oxidation and other oxidative species as well as prevention of inflammatory adhesion molecules in the vascular intima all of which are associated with atherogenesis. The initial clinical experience with IRNA was hampered by fairly high rates of flushing intolerance, but this has been largely overcome by the development of ERNA and attention to proper dosing and administration. Initial clinical trials of NA as monotherapy and in combination with other agents (statins, fibrates, and bile acid sequestrants) all showed significant lipid benefits. Two very large clinical trials (AIM-HIGH, and HPS-2 THRIVE) that were intended to confirm the benefits of NA/statin combined therapy had very disappointing results. Unfortunately, despite significant design flaws in these two studies, their results have led to widespread discontinuance of NA, both in combination with statins and even NA monotherapy. The real conclusion that seems supported by the two large clinical trials is that adding NA to statin treatment when a person is already at their LCL-C goal probably does not add benefit. But to disregard all of the prior positive NA studies and the fact that these large trials had serious design flaws is unfair judgment of NA. In fact, a 2013 meta-analysis of prior NA trials of both monotherapy and NA combined with other agents (included the Aim-High trial) showed that NA reduced risk of any CVD event by 34% and specifically major coronary event by 25% [48]. A similar meta-analysis of statin trials showed a 22 and 27% risk reduction for the same endpoints, respectively [49]. The obvious preference for statins when initialing lipid therapy is based on its effectiveness in lowering LDL-C, the prime lipid target in CVD risk reduction. But the NA trial with Endur-Acin showed that in a population with mild to moderate dyslipidemia, 50% or more of persons can reach their LDL-C goal with NA monotherapy and enjoy the additional lipid and non-lipid CVD benefits of NA therapy. Also, a recent study designed to evaluate the effects on atherogenic factors (lipid and non-lipid) when ERNA is added to statin therapy in MS patients showed an impressive array of positive benefits [50]. So, providers should continue to value its use in the many dyslipidemia patients who are appropriate for NA therapy and learn "how to do" NA for optimal results.

Author details

Joseph M. Keenan
Department of Family Medicine and Community Health, University of Minnesota, Minneapolis, Minnesota, USA

*Address all correspondence to: keena001@gmail.com

References

[1] Institute of Medicine. Dietary Reference Intakes for Thiamin, Riboflavin, Niacin, Vitamin B6, Folate, Vitamin B12, Pantothenic Acid, Biotin, and Choline. Washington, DC: The National Academies Press; 1998. pp. 123-149

[2] Bruckert E, Labreuche J, Amarenco P. Meta-analysis of the effect of nicotinic acid alone or in combination on cardiovascular events and atherosclerosis. Atherosclerosis. 2010;**210**(2):353-361

[3] Altshul R, Hoffer A, Stephen JD. Influence of nicotinic acid on serum cholesterol in man. Archives of Biochemistry and Biophysics. 1955;**54**:558-559

[4] Parsons WB Jr, Flinn JH. Reduction of serum cholesterol levels and beta-lipoprotein cholesterol levels by nicotinic acid. A.M.A. Archives of Internal Medicine. 1959;**103**(5):783-790

[5] Berge KG, Canner PL. Coronary drug project: Experience with niacin. Coronary drug project research group. European Journal of Clinical Pharmacology. 1991;**40**(Suppl 1): S49-S51

[6] Canner PL, Berge KG, Wenger NK, Stamler J, Friedman L, Prineas RJ, et al. Fifteen year mortality in coronary drug project patients: Long-term benefit with niacin. Journal of the American College of Cardiology. 1986;**8**(6):1245-1255

[7] Jellinger PS, Handelsman Y, Rosenblit PD, Bloomgarden ZT. American association of clinical endocrinologists and American college of endocrinology guidelines for management of dyslipidemia and prevention of cardiovascular disease. Endocrine Practice. 2017;**23**(Suppl 2):1-87

[8] Kamanna VS, Kashyap ML. Mechanism of action of niacin. The American Journal of Cardiology. 2008;**101**(8A):20B-26B. DOI: 10.1016/j.amjcard.2008.02.029

[9] Shehadah A, Chen J, Zacharek A, Cui Y, Ion M, Roberts C, et al. Niaspan treatment induces neuroprotection after stroke. Neurobiology of Disease. 2010;**40**(1):277-283

[10] Parsons WB Jr. Cholesterol Control Without Diet! The Niacin Solution

[11] Keenan JM, Fontaine PL, Wenz JB, Myers S, Huang ZQ. Niacin revisited. A randomized, controlled trial of wax-matrix sustained-release niacin in hypercholesterolemia. Archives of Internal Medicine. 1991;**151**(7):1424-1432

[12] Aronov DM. The role of nicotinic acid in the treatment of atherosclerosis and atherogenic dyslipidemia. Kliniceskaia Meditsina. 1996;**74**(9): 48-52 Review. Russian

[13] Keenan JM, Wenz JB, Ripsin CM, Huang Z, McCaffrey DJ. A clinical trial of oat bran and niacin in the treatment of hyperlipidemia. The Journal of Family Practice. 1992;**34**(3):313-319

[14] Goldberg RB, Bittner VA, Dunbar RL, et al. Effects of extended-release niacin added to simvastatin/ezetimibe on glucose and insulin values in AIM-HIGH. The American Journal of Medicine. 2016;**129**(7):753.E13-753.E22

[15] Canner PL, Furberg CD, McGovern ME. Benefits of niacin in patients with versus without the metabolic syndrome and healed myocardial infarction (from the coronary drug project). The American Journal of Cardiology. 2006;**97**(4):477-479. Epub 2005 Dec 21

[16] Shin D, Kongpakpaisarn K, Bohra C. Trends in the prevalence of metabolic syndrome and its components in the United States 2007-2014. International Journal of Cardiology. 2018;**259**:216-219

[17] Wilson PW, D'Agostino RB, Parise H, Sullivan L, Meigs JB. Metabolic syndrome as a precursor of cardiovascular disease and type 2 diabetes mellitus. Circulation. 2005;**112**(20):3066-3072. Epub 2005 Nov 7

[18] Kwasny C, Manuwald U, Kugler J, Rothe U. Systematic review of the epidemiology and natural history of the metabolic vascular syndrome and its coincidence with type 2 diabetes mellitus and cardiovascular diseases in different European countries. Hormone and Metabolic Research. 2018;**50**(3):201-208

[19] Chrysant SG, Ibrahim M. Niacin-ER/statin combination for the treatment of dyslipidemia: Focus on low high-density lipoprotein cholesterol. Journal of Clinical Hypertension (Greenwich, Conn.). 2006;**8**(7):493-499

[20] McKenney JM. Combination treatment with atorvastatin plus niacin provides effective control of complex dyslipidemias: A literature review. Postgraduate Medicine. 2012;**124**(1):7-20

[21] Cziraky MJ, Watson KE, Talbert RL. Targeting low HDL-cholesterol to decrease residual cardiovascular risk in the managed care setting. Managed Care Pharmacy. 2008;**14**(8 Suppl):S3-S28

[22] AIM-HIGH Investigators. The role of niacin in raising high-density lipoprotein cholesterol to reduce cardiovascular events in patients with atherosclerotic cardiovascular disease and optimally treated low-density lipoprotein cholesterol rationale and study design. The atherothrombosis intervention in metabolic syndrome with low HDL/high triglycerides: Impact on global health outcomes (AIM-HIGH). American Heart Journal. 2011;**161**(3):471-477

[23] The HPS2-THRIVE Collaborative Group. Effects of extended-release niacin with laropiprant in high-risk patients. The New England Journal of Medicine. 2014;**371**:203-212

[24] Guyton JR, Slee AE, Anderson T, Fleg JL, Goldberg RB, Kashyap ML, et al. Relationship of lipoproteins to cardiovascular events: The AIM-HIGH trial (atherothrombosis intervention in metabolic syndrome with low HDL/ high triglycerides and impact on global health outcomes). Journal of the American College of Cardiology. 2013;**62**(17):1580-1584

[25] Toth PP, Jones SR, Slee A, Fleg J, et al. Relationship between lipoprotein subfraction cholesterol and residual risk for cardiovascular outcomes: A post hoc analysis of the AIM-HIGH trial. Journal of Clinical Lipidology. 2018;**12**(3): 741-747.e11

[26] Superko HR, Zhao XQ, Hodis HN, Guyton JR. Niacin and heart disease prevention: Engraving its tombstone is a mistake. Journal of Clinical Lipidology. 2017;**11**(6):1309-1317

[27] HPS2-THRIVE Collaborative Group. HPS2-THRIVE randomized placebo-controlled trial in 25 673 high-risk patients of ER niacin/laropiprant: Trial design, pre-specified muscle and liver outcomes, and reasons for stopping study treatment. European Heart Journal. 2013;**34**(17):1279-1291

[28] Nayor M, Vasan RS. Recent update to the US cholesterol treatment guidelines: A comparison with international guidelines. Circulation. 2016;**133**(18):1795-1806

[29] Saxon DR, Eckel RH. Statin intolerance: A literature review and management strategies. Progress in

Cardiovascular Diseases. 2016; **59**(2):153-164

[30] Arrieta A, Page TF, Veledar E, Nasir K. Economic evaluation of PCSK9 inhibitors in reducing cardiovascular risk from health system and private payer perspectives. PLoS One. 2017;**12**(1):e0169761

[31] Lopez AD, Mathers CD, Ezzati M, Jamison DT, Murray CJ. Global and regional burden of disease and risk factors, 2001: Systematic analysis of population health data. Lancet. 2006;**367**(9524):1747-1757

[32] Pandya A, Sy S, Cho S, Weinstein MC, Gaziano TA. Cost-effectiveness of 10-year risk thresholds for initiation of statin therapy for primary prevention of cardiovascular disease. Journal of the American Medical Association. 2015;**314**:142-150

[33] Maki KC, Guyton JR, Orringer CE, Hamilton-Craig I, Alexander DD, Davidson MH. Triglyceride-lowering therapies reduce cardiovascular disease event risk in subjects with hypertriglyceridemia. Clinical Lipidology. 2016;**10**(4):905-914

[34] Sahebkar A, Reiner Ž, Simental-Mendía LE, Ferretti G, Cicero AF. Effect of extended-release niacin on plasma lipoprotein(a) levels: A systematic review and meta-analysis of randomized placebo-controlled trials. Metabolism. 2016;**65**(11):1664-1678

[35] Li M, Saeedi R, Rabkin SW, Frohlich J. Dramatic lowering of very high Lp(a) in response to niacin. Journal of Clinical Lipidology. 2014;**8**(4):448-450

[36] Knopp RH. Evaluating niacin in its various forms. The American Journal of Cardiology. 2000;**86**(12A):51L-56L

[37] Poon IO, Chow DS, Liang D. Dissolution profiles of nonprescription extended-release niacin and inositol niacinate products. American Journal of Health-System Pharmacy. 2006;**63**(21):2128-2134

[38] Vogt A, Kassner U, Hostalek U, Steinhagen-Thiessen E. NAUTILUS Study Group. Evaluation of the safety and tolerability of prolonged-release nicotinic acid in a usual care setting: The NAUTILUS study. Current Medical Research and Opinion. 2006;**22**(2):417-425

[39] Chaffman MO, Webster WB, Winiecki JT. Efficacy and safety evaluation of a large niacin therapeutic interchange program. The Annals of Pharmacotherapy. 2013;**47**(5):657-664

[40] Aronov DM, Keenan JM, Akhmedzhanov NM, Perova NV, Oganov RY, Kiseleva NY. Clinical trial of wax-matrix sustained-release niacin in a Russian population with hypercholesterolemia. Archives of Family Medicine. 1996;**5**(10):567-575

[41] Keenan JM. Wax-matrix extended-release niacin vs inositol hexanicotinate: A comparison of wax-matrix, extended-release niacin to inositol hexanicotinate "no-flush" niacin in persons with mild to moderate dyslipidemia. Journal of Clinical Lipidology. 2013;7(1):14-23

[42] Keenan JM, Bae CY, Fontaine PL, Wenz JB, Myers S, Huang ZQ, et al. Treatment of hypercholesterolemia: Comparison of younger versus older patients using wax-matrix sustained-release niacin. Journal of the American Geriatrics Society. 1992;**40**(1):12-18

[43] Knopp RH, Retzlaff BM, Fish B, Dowdy A, Twaddell B, Nguyen T, et al. The SLIM study: Slo-Niacin® and atorvastatin treatment of lipoproteins and inflammatory markers in combined hyperlipidemia. Journal of Clinical Lipidology. 2009;**3**(3):167-178

[44] Knopp RH, Alagona P, Davidson M, et al. Equivalent efficacy of a time-release form of niacin (Niaspan) given once-a-night versus plain niacin

in the management of hyperlipidemia. Metabolism. 1998;**47**:1097-1104

[45] Morgan JM, Capuzzi DM, Guyton JR, Centor RM, Goldberg R, Robbins DC, et al. Treatment effect of Niaspan, a controlled-release niacin, in patients with hypercholesterolemia: A placebo-controlled trial. Journal of Cardiovascular Pharmacology and Therapeutics. 1996;**1**(3):195-202

[46] Vogt A, Kassner U, Hostalek U, Steinhagen-Thiessen E. Prolonged-release nicotinic acid for the management of dyslipidemia: An update including results from the NAUTILUS study. Vascular Health and Risk Management. 2007;**3**(4):467-479

[47] Villines TC, Stanek EJ, Devine PJ, Turco M, Miller M, Weissman NJ, et al. The ARBITER 6-HALTS trial (arterial biology for the investigation of the treatment effects of reducing cholesterol 6-HDL and LDL treatment strategies in atherosclerosis): Final results and the impact of medication adherence, dose, and treatment duration. Journal of the American College of Cardiology. 2010;**55**(24):2721-2726

[48] Lavigne PM, Karas RH. The current state of niacin in cardiovascular disease prevention: A systematic review and meta-regression. Journal of the American College of Cardiology. 2013;**61**(4):440-446

[49] Baigent C, Blackwell L, Emberson J, et al. Efficacy and safety of more intensive lowering of LDL cholesterol: A meta-analysis of data from 170,000 participants in 26 randomized trials. Lancet. 2010;**376**:1670-1681

[50] Adiels M, Chapman MJ, Robillard P, et al. Niacin action in the atherogenic mixed dyslipidemia of metabolic syndrome: Insights from metabolic biomarker profiling and network analysis. Journal of Clinical Lipidology. 2018;**12**:810-821

Chapter 8

Novel Therapies for Dyslipidemia

Olta Tafaj Reddy

Abstract

Multiple studies have shown a strong correlation between low-density lipoprotein cholesterol (LDL-C) concentration and development as well as progression of atherosclerosis and cardiovascular disorders. Thus, the decrease of the LDL-C burden through lifestyle modification and/or pharmacological interventions unanimously demonstrated a decrease in cardiovascular events and mortality. To date, statins are considered the cornerstone of lipid-lowering therapy. The Cholesterol Treatment Trialists' (CTT) Collaboration has shown consistency of treatment benefits across a wide patient population. However, new data are now revealing that a considerate patient population failed to achieve lipid goals solely on statins and a significant percentage cannot tolerate treatment. Therefore, extensive work has recently been done in generating novel LDL-C-lowering agents that would act through mechanisms different from statins. Among others, monoclonal antibodies to protein convertase subtilisin/kexin type 9 (PCSK9) and ezetimibe seem particularly promising. Both PCSK9 monoclonal antibodies and ezetimibe have shown to be well tolerated and very effective at lowering LDL-C.

Keywords: dyslipidemia, PCSK9 inhibitors, ezetimibe, LDL-C

1. Introduction

Cardiovascular disease (CVD), which includes coronary heart disease (CHD) and strokes, is considered as a number one cause of morbidity and mortality worldwide. Together with hypertension, dyslipidemia is among the most prevalent risk factors leading to CVD. Thus, treatment of dyslipidemia is crucial in reducing CVD events and the morbidity and mortality associated with them. Studies in the last decade have confirmed a causal relationship between low-density lipoprotein cholesterol (LDL-C) and the risk of atherosclerotic cardiovascular diseases (ASCVD) [1]. LDL-C can be lowered by diet restriction and lifestyle changes or by various lipid-lowering therapies, among which statins (3-hydroxy-3-methylglutaryl-coenzyme A [HMG-CoA] reductase inhibitors) are currently considered the cornerstone medication. Based on the 2018 guidelines published by the American College of Cardiology (ACC) and the American Heart Association (AHA), multiple recommendations have been made for patients with or at risk of developing cardiovascular disease [2].

Under certain circumstances, non-statin medications like ezetimibe and PCSK9 inhibitors are found to be useful particularly in combination with statin therapy. Clinical trials pertaining to these novel therapies have shown great benefits with significant LDL-C-lowering potential and decrease in cardiovascular risk. These agents are generally well tolerated, but long-term safety and cost remain to be proven.

2. PCSK9 inhibitors as cholesterol-lowering therapy

2.1 Genetics behind the discovery of PCSK9 inhibitors

PCSK9 gene was initially discovered as part of a search for members of the protein convertase family of serine proteases [3]. It was initially named as neural apoptosis-regulated convertase-1 (NARC1) due to its upregulation in apoptosis of primary cultures of cerebellar neurons. Subsequent studies classified it as a member of the proteinase K family of subtilases, and it was renamed as (proprotein convertase subtilisin/kexin type 9 (PCSK9)). The gene mapped to chromosome 1p32 comprises 12 exons, and it is translated into a protein of 692 amino acids (NM-174936.3) and is mainly expressed in the liver [3]. Interestingly, the gene coding for PCSK9 coincides with a region linked to dominant inheritance of hypercholesterolemia in American and French families who had no mutations in either LDL-R or APOB genes [4, 5]. Loss-of-function mutations in the later are the two main culprits that comprise 99% of cases with familial hypercholesterolemia (FH). Further genetic analysis of these index families identified a few rare heterozygous missense mutations in PCSK9 gene, all coinciding with hypercholesterolemia [6]. Thus, PCSK9 is now recognized as the third gene causing FH and currently accounts for <1% of FH cases [7].

A crucial step in further understanding the role of this gene in cholesterol metabolism was achieved by Maxwell and Breslow, who showed that transgenic overexpression of PCSK9 in mice caused a FH-like phenotype due to increased intracellular degradation of the LDL-receptor (LDL-R) [8, 9]. This observation shed light into the physiological implication of PCSK9 gene in the lipid metabolism and dyslipidemia. It became clear that gain-of-function rather than loss-of-function mutations in PCSK9 lead to hypercholesterolemia. In the last decade, many disease-causing mutations, occurring in various domains of the protein and leading to either increased transcription or impaired autocatalysis, have confirmed the above findings [10–13].

It was not until 2005 when studies in individuals with extremely low LDL-C levels revealed some PCSK9 coding variants that were not seen in individuals with high levels of LDL-C. Some of these variants encoded truncated version of the protein that was clearly predicted to cause loss-of-function of PCSK9 [14, 15]. Mendelian randomization experiments clearly revealed that individuals with PCSK9 loss-of-function variants had lifelong depressed LDL-C levels as well as reduced ASCVD risk [16]. In these initial studies, of 3363 blacks, 2.6% carried heterozygous PCSK9 nonsense variants and were associated with 28 and 88% reductions in LDL-C and ASCVD risk, respectively. Of the 9524 white subjects examined, 3.2% had a PCSK9 mutation and were associated with 15 and 47% reductions in LDL-C and ASCVD risk, respectively. The above results were then confirmed in subsequent larger cohort studies [17, 18].

Taken together, the findings in either gain-of-function or loss-of-function mutations in PCSK9 gene have provided very strong evidence for the potential pharmacological use of targeted reduction of PCSK9 protein. Additionally, studies of complete human knockouts of PCSK9 (biallelic loss-of-function mutations) revealed only isolated decreased LDL-C levels with no deleterious health complications [19, 20]. This supports the potential safety of pharmacologically targeting PCSK9. However, it is worth mentioning that carriers of PCSK9 loss-of-function mutations showed an increased risk of developing type 2 diabetes mellitus (T2DM) [21, 22]. This finding would suggest that a similar side effect may be encountered in potential pharmacological inhibitors of PCSK9 (an increase of T2DM has been reported in statin drugs) [23]. However, no such association was found in clinical trials with human monoclonal anti-PCSK9 [24]. An increased risk of T2DM was also observed in a phenome-wide association study performed in >337,000 individuals with PCSK9 p.R46L mutation [25]. The same mutation was found to have a protective effect on hyperlipidemia, coronary heart disease (CHD), ischemic stroke, and cerebral infarction. No association with cataracts, heart failure, atrial fibrillation, or cognitive dysfunction was reported.

2.2 Mechanism of action of PCSK9 protein

PCSK9 is a serine protease involved in cholesterol metabolism. In the liver, it binds to the LDL-receptor (LDL-R), inducing intracellular degradation, thus reducing serum LDL clearance. Generally, PCSK9 molecule is absent allowing repeated recycling of the LDL-R receptor. One study also suggests that intracellular PCSK9 may be recycled so that a single molecule might contribute multiple times to receptor degradation [26]. Under physiological conditions, PCSK9 expression is very low compared to LDL-R, thus allowing continuous recycling of the receptor (**Figure 1A**). In the case of low intracellular levels of cholesterol, both LDL-R and PCSK9 are transcribed (**Figure 1B**). Once secreted in the plasma, PCSK9 serves as one of the many potential ligands for LDL-R. After endocytosis, LDL-R, LDL particle, and PCSK9 enter the lysosome. Once inside the lysosome, the LDL particle is degraded, whereas the LDL-R attached to PCSK9 fails to exit the lysosome, where it gets degraded and can no longer be recycled (**Figure 1B**) [10, 27, 28]. Using this intricate mechanism, PCSK9 would prevent overexpression of LDL-R and thus increase the intracellular cholesterol levels. On the other hand, in patients with elevated cholesterol levels, administering PCSK9 monoclonal antibodies would neutralize the PCSK9 molecules floating in the plasma, thus increasing LDL-R recycling and surface LDL-R (**Figure 1C**).

To better understand the action of PCSK9 inhibitors, we can correlate it with the pharmacological action of HMG-CoA reductase inhibitors (statins). Cholesterol is mainly synthetized in the liver via the mevalonate pathway, with HMG-CoA reductase being the rate-limiting enzyme in the process. The decrease in the intracellular cholesterol in the liver is sensed by sterol regulatory element-binding protein 2 (SREBP2) which then increases the production of HMG-CoA reductase to promote the intracellular synthesis of cholesterol as well as increase LDL-R and PCSK9 levels. As a result, statins will (1) decrease intracellular cholesterol production, (2) increase LDL-R expression on the hepatocytes, and (3) increase PCSK9 levels. This

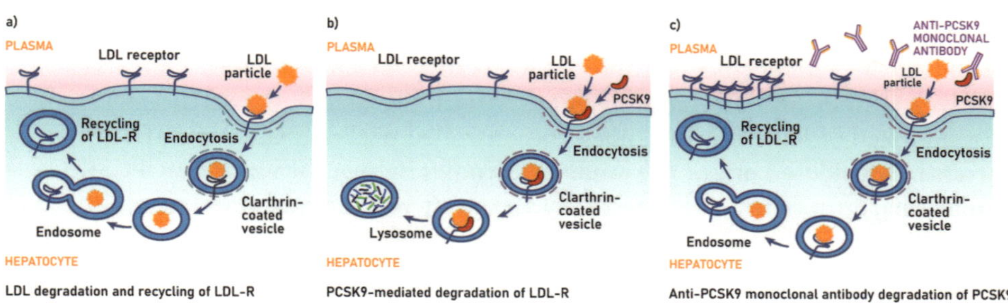

Figure 1.
Under physiological conditions, PCSK9 expression is very low compared to LDL-R, thus allowing continuous recycling of the receptor (a). In the case of low intracellular levels of cholesterol, both LDL-R and PCSK9 are transcribed (b). In patients with elevated cholesterol levels, administering PCSK9 monoclonal antibodies would neutralize the PCSK9 molecules floating in the plasma, thus increasing LDL-R recycling and surface LDL-R (c).

can explain why addition of anti-PCSK9 monoclonal antibodies can accentuate the lipid-lowering effect of statins.

2.3 Therapeutic rationale for PCSK9 inhibitors

Currently, statins are the first-choice agents to reduce high blood cholesterol which is considered one of the main risk factors for cardiovascular disease (CVD). Cholesterol Treatment Trialists' (CTT) Collaboration as well as other clinical trials showed that primary prevention with statins reduced all-cause mortality, reduced combined fatal and nonfatal stroke, reduced revascularization rate, and improved patient quality of life [29, 30]. Statin prescription is not associated with serious harm and is considered to be cost-effective [31]. That said, in the last decade, many patients have reported more and more severe side effects particularly with high-intensity statin therapy [32]. Additionally, certain patient populations (familial hypercholesterolemia) are at particular high risk for cardiovascular events. The risk can be attributed to the complexity of the underlying disease, and sole treatment with statins may be insufficient.

Familial hypercholesterolemia: Familial hypercholesterolemia (FH) is a complex genetic disorder characterized by high LDL-C levels and early incidence of ASCVD [33]. There are two forms of FH: a heterozygous and homozygous one with a prevalence of 1 in 250 and 1 in 250,000, respectively [34]. The disorder is characterized by high-serum LDL-C concentration, xanthomas including Achilles tendon thickening, and premature coronary artery disease (CAD). In FH patients, the prevalence of CAD is extremely high, and its age of onset is 15–20 years earlier than usual. Thus, early diagnosis and appropriate treatment are crucial.

Statin intolerance: Statin intolerance is defined as an inability to take statin because of reported side effects. It is classified as complete (inability to tolerate any statin at any dose) or partial (inability to tolerate high doses of statin). The most common reported adverse effect is muscle pain due to myopathy and rhabdomyolysis in severe cases. Though rare, rhabdomyolysis can be serious if not detected and treated early. An increased risk of type 2 diabetes has also been reported, particularly with high-dose statins [35]. Two recent meta-analyses observed a 9% increased risk for incident diabetes associated with statin therapy, with little heterogeneity between studies. Hemorrhagic stroke also appears to be increased by statin therapy, although estimates are imprecise. However, overall stroke events were reduced, indicating a net benefit.

2.4 Anti-PCSK9 monoclonal antibodies and the cardiovascular outcome studies

Multiple studies were performed to investigate the cardiovascular effect of the anti-PCSK9 monoclonal antibodies. The Further Cardiovascular Outcomes Research with PCSK9 Inhibition in Subjects with Elevated Risk (FOURIER) trial, a randomized, double-blinded, placebo-controlled trial published in 2017, is currently considered one of the landmark studies in the efficacy of anti-PCSK9 monoclonal antibodies [36]. The aim of the study was to understand whether evolocumab (anti-PCSK9 monoclonal antibody) which lowers LDL-C levels by 69% can prevent cardiovascular events. This trial included 27,564 patients with atherosclerotic cardiovascular disease and LDL-C levels of ≥70 mg/dl while on maximally tolerated statin therapy. Patients were then randomly assigned to either evolocumab (140 mg every 2 weeks or 429 mg monthly) or placebo. The primary end point of the study was the composite of cardiovascular death, myocardial infarction, stroke, hospitalization for unstable angina, or coronary revascularization. The secondary end point was the composite of cardiovascular death, myocardial infarction, or stroke. The median duration of follow-up was 2.2 years. Inhibition of PCSK9 with evolocumab on a background of statin therapy lowered LDL-C levels to a median of 30 mg/dl. Addition of evolocumab to statin therapy significantly reduces the risk of cardiovascular events, with a 15% reduction risk of primary composite and a 20% reduction risk of the secondary composite outcomes. Based on this study, PCSK9 inhibitor therapy should be considered for ASCVD risk reduction in patients with stable ASCVD, particularly in those with additional risk factors, on maximally tolerated statin therapy, with on-treatment LDL-C ≥70 mg/dl or non-HDL-C ≥100 mg/dl. In the same FOURIER trial, similar recommendations but with a lower level of evidence can also be applicable to patients with progressive ASCVD (additional diagnosis of MI or nonhemorrhagic stroke).

2.5 Anti-PCSK9 monoclonal antibodies in patients with statin intolerance

There is currently no universally accepted definition for statin intolerance. Previous studies have confirmed statin-related muscle side effects; however more needs to be done to accurately address the issue. That said, statin intolerance in individuals with a history of CVD is a challenge to a clinician. According to the latest National Lipid Association (NLA) recommendations, PCSK9 inhibitors may be considered to reduce LDL-C in selected very-high-risk patients who are classified as statin-intolerant, in the presence of additional LDL-C-lowering therapies [37]. The quality of evidence for such a recommendation is low.

2.6 Anti-PCSK9 monoclonal antibodies in patients with severe hypercholesterolemia

Severe hypercholesterolemia is defined as LDL-C ≥190 mg/dl. The majority of these patients have polygenic hypercholesterolemia attributed to multiple, undefined genetic factors. Familial hypercholesterolemia (both heterozygous and homozygous) is due to defined mutations yet less commonly encountered. Regardless of the etiology, long-term risk for cardiovascular diseases in all these patients is very high. However, studies have shown that particularly patients with clinically defined FH have a greater risk for cardiovascular events despite being on maximum dose of statins. Studies in patients with heterozygous familial hypercholesterolemia who received PCSK9 inhibitors (either alirocumab or evolocumab) revealed significant additional LDL-C reduction.

Based on the current data, the National Lipid Association is recommending addition of PCSK9 inhibitors in patients with LDL-C ≥190 mg/dl with additional risk factors or genetic confirmation of FH on maximally tolerated statin ± ezetimibe.

2.7 Intravascular ultrasound trial

In order to determine the effects of PCSK9 inhibitors (evolocumab) on progression of coronary atherosclerosis in statin-treated patients, the Global Assessment of Plaque Regression with a PCSK9 Antibody as Measured by Intravascular Ultrasound (GLAGOV) multicenter, double-blind, placebo-controlled, randomized clinical trial was conducted [38]. In this trial 968 patients with angiographic coronary disease were studied. These patients were randomized to receive monthly 420 mg evolocumab or placebo via subcutaneous injection for 76 weeks, in addition to moderate- or high-intensity statins. In this trial, the primary efficacy was the change in percent atheroma volume from baseline to week 78, measured by serial intravascular ultrasonography (IVUS) imaging. Secondary efficacy was measured in normalized total atheroma volume and patients demonstrating plaque regression. Interestingly, IVUS showed atherosclerosis regression during 18 months of therapy in patients treated with the combination of evolocumab and statins and absence of regression in patients treated with statin alone. Additionally, the evolocumab group showed a significant reduction in percent atheroma volume as well as total atheroma volume (−0.95%, $p < 0.01$, between group difference, −4.9 mm^3, $p < 0.01$, respectively). Taken together, PCSK9 inhibitors produce additional benefits on coronary disease progression in statin-treated patients.

2.8 Efficacy and safety of anti-PCSK9 monoclonal antibodies

The most recent study to evaluate the effects of alirocumab on the occurrence of cardiovascular events in patients who have experienced an acute coronary syndrome (ODYSSEY OUTCOMES) suggested a reduction in mortality with alirocumab in patients after acute coronary syndrome [39].Based on the results from multiple trials, alirocumab reduced the risk of all-cause mortality: 6 fewer deaths per 1000 patients treated (RR, 0.82; 95% CI 0.72–0.95). No reduction in cardiovascular mortality was observed (RR, 0.87; 95% CI, 0.73–1.02) [40]. On the other hand, trials of evolocumab did not show a reduction in either all-cause or cardiovascular mortality (RR, 0.91; 95% CI, 0.57–1.44 and RR, 1.04; 95% CI, 0.88–1.24, respectively). Taken together, PCSK9 inhibitors did not reduce the risk of all-cause or cardiovascular mortality.

Both alirocumab and evolocumab reduced the risk of myocardial infarction, stroke, and coronary revascularization. Alirocumab, but not evolocumab, reduced stable angina hospitalization, and neither drug reduced heart failure.

Regarding the safety of anti-PCSK9 monoclonal antibodies (alirocumab and evolocumab), all phase 2 and 3 studies have demonstrated excellent safety profile [41]. The most commonly reported adverse effect has been injection site reaction [42]. As part of the safety analysis, fat-soluble vitamin concentrations (A, D, E, K) were measured. Compared to placebo, no change in the levels of any of these vitamins was reported. Additionally, no increase in neurocognitive events, new-onset or worsening diabetes, muscle-related events, or myalgia has been noted [43].

Bococizumab has been excluded from most of these studies as the drug is no longer available after the cessation of development by the manufacturer due to high rates of neutralizing antibody formation and subsequent loss of therapeutic efficacy (SPIRE trial) [44].

3. Ezetimibe as cholesterol-lowering therapy

Since the early 1990s when statins were initially introduced, several large clinical trials have highlighted the benefits of their use with beneficial effects above and beyond lipid lowering [45]. Statins are currently the cornerstone of hyperlipidemia treatment. However, due to safety concerning high-dose therapy as well as residual risk of CVD especially in high-risk patients, additional lipid-modifying therapies have emerged in the last decades.

Ezetimibe reduces absorption of cholesterol from the brush border of the small intestine by targeting the Niemann-Pick C1-like 1 (NPC1L1) protein (**Figure 2**) [46, 47]. Genetic studies have shown that polymorphisms affecting NPC1L1 are associated with lower levels of LDL cholesterol and a lower risk of cardiovascular diseases [48]. A decrease in cholesterol absorption results in a decrease of total cholesterol, triglycerides, and LDL cholesterol and an increase in HDL cholesterol.

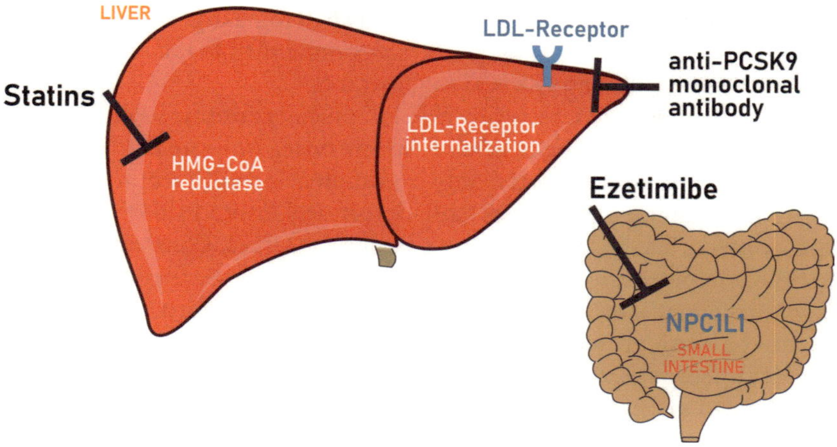

Figure 2.
Ezetimibe reduces absorption of cholesterol from the brush border of the small intestine by targeting the Niemann-Pick C1-like 1 (NPC1L1) protein. In the liver, HMG-CoA reductase (statins) promotes the intracellular synthesis of cholesterol as well as increases LDL-R and PCKS9 levels. PCSK9 monoclonal antibodies would neutralize the PCSK9 molecules floating in the plasma, thus increasing LDL-R recycling and surface LDL-R in the liver.

It was FDA-approved in 2002 as an agent to treat people with hyperlipidemia. Ezetimibe given as monotherapy leads to an LDL reduction of approximately 20%. When added to statins, ezetimibe reduces LDL cholesterol levels by an additional 23–24% on average [49, 50]. The Improved Reduction of Outcomes: Vytorin Efficacy International Trial (IMPROVE-IT) was then conducted to understand if further lowering of the LDL-C levels by statin-ezetimibe dual therapy leads to clinical benefit [51]. In this trial they studied the effect of ezetimibe combined with simvastatin, as compared with that of simvastatin alone, in stable patients who had an acute coronary syndrome and whose LDL cholesterol values were within the guideline recommendations. The primary end points were death from cardiovascular disease, a major coronary event, or nonfatal stroke, assessed from the time of randomization until the first occurrence of one of the events. The combination of simvastatin and ezetimibe resulted in additional lowering of LDL-C levels as well as lower risk of cardiovascular event. A reduction of cholesterol levels of 12.8 mg per deciliter correlated with a proportionally 7.2% lower rate of major vascular events, providing further evidence for a relationship between lower lipid and improved outcomes.

Multiple statin trials including the CTT collaboration have shown clinical benefits when LDL cholesterol was lowered to progressively lower levels. It was on the basis of these trials that a LDL-C of <70 mg per deciliter has been recommended for patients with acute coronary syndrome. Data from the IMPROVE-IT trial support the previous finding and show a direct evidence between further lipid lowering and improved outcomes [51]. Additionally, this trial provides evidence, for the first time, that a non-statin lipid-lowering agent can reduce cardiovascular risk by lowering LDL-C and that statins are not the only beneficiary drugs in hyperlipidemia. The American College of Cardiology recommends consideration of ezetimibe therapy in addition to maximally tolerated statin therapy for both primary and secondary prevention in patients who have not achieved target reduction in their LDL-C by maximally tolerated statin therapy alone.

3.1 Administration, side effects, and contraindications of ezetimibe

Ezetimibe is currently marketed as a monotherapy under the trade name of Zetia, as well as in combination with a statin such as Vytorin and Liptruzet. It has a half-life of 22 hours, and it can be administered at 10 mg daily. It can be taken at the same time as fenofibrates or statins, but it is recommended to take it at least 2 hours before or 4 hours after taking bile acid sequestrants.

Based on current studies, very few side effects to ezetimibe have been reported, most common being headache, runny nose, and sore throat [52]. Rhabdomyolysis has been reported only in combination with statin therapy and rarely with monotherapy. Due to its daily dosing and limited side effects, ezetimibe is considered a safer drug with no compliance issues. Contraindications to its use include hypersensitivity to possible ingredients of the formulation. It is not recommended in patients with moderate to severe hepatic impairment but can be administered in patients with renal impairment without any need for dose adjustment. Liver function tests need to be performed only if it is administered with a statin. It is worth mentioning that patients taking ezetimibe with cyclosporine are at an increased risk of ezetimibe toxicity as it can result in 2.3–12-fold increase in exposure [53]. In these cases, cyclosporine concentrations should be closely monitored.

3.2 Ezetimibe versus anti-PCSK9 monoclonal inhibitor (evolocumab) as add-on therapy for secondary prevention of cardiovascular events

When results from trials of ezetimibe (IMPROVE-IT) and PCSK9 inhibitors (FOURIER RCT) are compared in regard to secondary prevention of cardiovascular events in patients with ASCVD and type 2 diabetes, evolocumab (PCSK9 inhibitor) seems to be more effective [54]. Interestingly, as of December 2018, the annual cost of evolocumab is $6540 and $88 for ezetimibe. From a healthcare cost standpoint, ezetimibe has a significantly lower cost and may be considered a preferred add-on therapy for these patients. The difference in avoiding cardiovascular events between the two therapies is negligible compared with the significant difference in the drug costs. However, a randomized controlled trial (RCT) comparing evolocumab and ezetimibe would be necessary to evaluate and compare the effectiveness of these two drugs. Additionally, long-term effects of these novel drugs in reducing the cardiovascular events in patients with ASCVD and type 2 diabetes will be needed.

4. Conclusions

Dyslipidemia is a major risk factor for both fatal and nonfatal CVD. Lowering cholesterol levels particularly LDL-C, through lifestyle modifications as well as pharmacological interventions, is crucial for CVD risk reduction. Currently, statins are the cornerstone medication for treatment and primary prevention of hypercholesterolemia. Studies have shown that benefits from statins outweigh any possible adverse effects. However, as the intensity of statin therapy increases, intolerance to their use becomes more prominent. Additionally, high-risk patients on maximally tolerated statins may benefit from novel LDL-C-lowering therapies. Clinical trials have provided evidence that these novel drugs such as PCSK9 inhibitors or ezetimibe can successfully lower LDL-C in levels and contribute in lowering cardiovascular events in high-risk patients with elevated LDL-C on maximally tolerated statins. Both ezetimibe and PCSK9 inhibitors have demonstrated a modest absolute ASCVD risk reduction and good safety profiles. However, given cost considerations particularly for PCSK9 inhibitors, healthcare providers will need to carefully consider the subgroup of patients benefiting the most from their use.

Conflict of interest

The author declares no conflict of interest.

Author details

Olta Tafaj Reddy
Department of Medicine, SUNY Downstate Medical Center, Brooklyn, NY, USA

*Address all correspondence to: olta.tafaj-reddy@downstate.edu

References

[1] Ference BA et al. Low-density lipoproteins cause atherosclerotic cardiovascular disease. 1. Evidence from genetic, epidemiologic, and clinical studies. A consensus statement from the European Atherosclerosis Society Consensus Panel. European Heart Journal. 2017;**38**(32):2459-2472

[2] Grundy SM, et al. AHA/ACC/AACVPR/AAPA/ABC/ACPM/ADA/AGS/APhA/ASPC/NLA/PCNA Guideline on the Management of Blood Cholesterol: A Report of the American College of Cardiology/American Heart Association Task Force on Clinical Practice Guidelines. Circulation 2018. 2019;**139**(25):e1082-e1143

[3] Seidah NG et al. The secretory proprotein convertase neural apoptosis-regulated convertase 1 (NARC-1): Liver regeneration and neuronal differentiation. Proceedings of the National Academy of Sciences of the United States of America. 2003;**100**(3):928-933

[4] Varret M et al. A third major locus for autosomal dominant hypercholesterolemia maps to 1p34.1-p32. American Journal of Human Genetics. 1999;**64**(5):1378-1387

[5] Hunt SC et al. Genetic localization to chromosome 1p32 of the third locus for familial hypercholesterolemia in a Utah kindred. Arteriosclerosis, Thrombosis, and Vascular Biology. 2000;**20**(4):1089-1093

[6] Abifadel M et al. Mutations in PCSK9 cause autosomal dominant hypercholesterolemia. Nature Genetics. 2003;**34**(2):154-156

[7] Nordestgaard BG et al. Familial hypercholesterolaemia is underdiagnosed and undertreated in the general population: Guidance for clinicians to prevent coronary heart disease: Consensus statement of the European atherosclerosis society. European Heart Journal. 2013;**34**(45):3478-390a

[8] Maxwell KN, Fisher EA, Breslow JL. Overexpression of PCSK9 accelerates the degradation of the LDLR in a post-endoplasmic reticulum compartment. Proceedings of the National Academy of Sciences of the United States of America. 2005;**102**(6):2069-2074

[9] Maxwell KN, Breslow JL. Adenoviral-mediated expression of PCSK9 in mice results in a low-density lipoprotein receptor knockout phenotype. Proceedings of the National Academy of Sciences of the United States of America. 2004;**101**(18):7100-7105

[10] Burke AC et al. PCSK9: Regulation and target for drug development for dyslipidemia. Annual Review of Pharmacology and Toxicology. 2017;**57**:223-244

[11] Seidah NG et al. The proprotein convertases in hypercholesterolemia and cardiovascular diseases: Emphasis on proprotein convertase subtilisin/kexin 9. Pharmacological Reviews. 2017;**69**(1):33-52

[12] Dron JS, Hegele RA. Complexity of mechanisms among human proprotein convertase subtilisin-kexin type 9 variants. Current Opinion in Lipidology. 2017;**28**(2):161-169

[13] Iacocca MA et al. Whole-gene duplication of PCSK9 as a novel genetic mechanism for severe familial hypercholesterolemia. The Canadian Journal of Cardiology. 2018;**34**(10):1316-1324

[14] Cohen J et al. Low LDL cholesterol in individuals of African descent

resulting from frequent nonsense mutations in PCSK9. Nature Genetics. 2005;**37**(2):161-165

[15] Kotowski IK et al. A spectrum of PCSK9 alleles contributes to plasma levels of low-density lipoprotein cholesterol. American Journal of Human Genetics. 2006;**78**(3):410-422

[16] Cohen JC et al. Sequence variations in PCSK9, low LDL, and protection against coronary heart disease. The New England Journal of Medicine. 2006;**354**(12):1264-1272

[17] Kent ST et al. PCSK9 loss-of-function variants, low-density lipoprotein cholesterol, and risk of coronary heart disease and stroke: Data from 9 studies of blacks and whites. Circulation. Cardiovascular Genetics. 2017;**10**(4):e001632

[18] Benn M et al. PCSK9 R46L, low-density lipoprotein cholesterol levels, and risk of ischemic heart disease: 3 independent studies and meta-analyses. Journal of the American College of Cardiology. 2010;**55**(25):2833-2842

[19] Zhao Z et al. Molecular characterization of loss-of-function mutations in PCSK9 and identification of a compound heterozygote. American Journal of Human Genetics. 2006;**79**(3):514-523

[20] Hooper AJ et al. The C679X mutation in PCSK9 is present and lowers blood cholesterol in a southern African population. Atherosclerosis. 2007;**193**(2):445-448

[21] Schmidt AF et al. PCSK9 genetic variants and risk of type 2 diabetes: A mendelian randomisation study. The Lancet Diabetes and Endocrinology. 2017;**5**(2):97-105

[22] Ference BA et al. Variation in PCSK9 and HMGCR and risk of cardiovascular disease and diabetes. The New England Journal of Medicine. 2016;**375**(22):2144-2153

[23] Preiss D, Sattar N. Statins and the risk of new-onset diabetes: A review of recent evidence. Current Opinion in Lipidology. 2011;**22**(6):460-466

[24] Cao YX et al. Effect of proprotein convertase subtilisin/kexin type 9 (PCSK9) monoclonal antibodies on new-onset diabetes mellitus and glucose metabolism: A systematic review and meta-analysis. Diabetes, Obesity & Metabolism. 2018;**20**(6):1391-1398

[25] Rao AS et al. Large-scale phenome-wide association study of PCSK9 variants demonstrates protection against ischemic stroke. Circulation: Genomic and Precision Medicine. 2018;**11**(7):e002162

[26] Rosenson RS et al. The evolving future of PCSK9 inhibitors. Journal of the American College of Cardiology. 2018;**72**(3):314-329

[27] Seidah NG. New developments in proprotein convertase subtilisin-kexin 9's biology and clinical implications. Current Opinion in Lipidology. 2016;**27**(3):274-281

[28] Rosenson RS, Hegele RA, Koenig W. Cholesterol-lowering agents. Circulation Research. 2019;**124**(3):364-385

[29] Cholesterol Treatment Trialists, C et al. Efficacy and safety of more intensive lowering of LDL cholesterol: A meta-analysis of data from 170,000 participants in 26 randomised trials. Lancet. 2010;**376**(9753):1670-1681

[30] Cholesterol Treatment Trialists, C et al. Efficacy and safety of LDL-lowering therapy among men and women: Meta-analysis of individual data from 174,000 participants in 27 randomised trials. Lancet. 2015;**385**(9976):1397-1405

[31] Cholesterol Treatment Trialists, C. Efficacy and safety of statin therapy in older people: A meta-analysis of individual participant data from 28 randomised controlled trials. Lancet. 2019;**393**(10170):407-415

[32] Taylor F et al. Statins for the primary prevention of cardiovascular disease. The Cochrane Database of Systematic Reviews. 2013;(1):CD004816. DOI: 10.1002/14651858.CD004816.pub5. Review

[33] Defesche JC et al. Familial hypercholesterolaemia. Nature Reviews. Disease Primers. 2017;**3**:17093

[34] Akioyamen LE et al. Estimating the prevalence of heterozygous familial hypercholesterolaemia: A systematic review and meta-analysis. BMJ Open. 2017;7(9):e016461

[35] Kamran H et al. Statins and new-onset diabetes in cardiovascular and kidney disease cohorts: A meta-analysis. Cardiorenal Medicine. 2018;**8**(2):105-112

[36] Sabatine MS et al. Evolocumab and clinical outcomes in patients with cardiovascular disease. The New England Journal of Medicine. 2017;**376**(18):1713-1722

[37] Orringer CE et al. Update on the use of PCSK9 inhibitors in adults: Recommendations from an expert panel of the National Lipid Association. Journal of Clinical Lipidology. 2017;**11**(4):880-890

[38] Puri R et al. Impact of PCSK9 inhibition on coronary atheroma progression: Rationale and design of global assessment of plaque regression with a PCSK9 antibody as measured by intravascular ultrasound (GLAGOV). American Heart Journal. 2016;**176**:83-92

[39] Schwartz GG et al. Alirocumab and cardiovascular outcomes after acute coronary syndrome. The New England Journal of Medicine. 2018;**379**(22):2097-2107

[40] Turgeon RD et al. Cardiovascular efficacy and safety of PCSK9 inhibitors: Systematic review and meta-analysis including the ODYSSEY OUTCOMES trial. Canadian Journal of Cardiology. 2018;**34**(12):1600-1605

[41] Robinson JG et al. Safety of very low low-density lipoprotein cholesterol levels with alirocumab: Pooled data from randomized trials. Journal of the American College of Cardiology. 2017;**69**(5):471-482

[42] Robinson JG et al. Efficacy and safety of alirocumab in reducing lipids and cardiovascular events. New England Journal of Medicine. 2015;**372**(16):1489-1499

[43] Giugliano RP, Sabatine MS, Ott BR. Cognitive function in a randomized trial of evolocumab. New England Journal of Medicine. 2017;**377**(20):1997

[44] Ridker PM et al. Lipid-reduction variability and antidrug-antibody formation with bococizumab. New England Journal of Medicine. 2017;**376**(16):1517-1526

[45] McFarlane SI et al. Clinical review 145: Pleiotropic effects of statins: Lipid reduction and beyond. The Journal of Clinical Endocrinology & Metabolism. 2002;**87**(4):1451-1458

[46] Sudhop T et al. Inhibition of intestinal cholesterol absorption by ezetimibe in humans. Circulation. 2002;**106**(15):1943-1948

[47] Kosoglou T et al. Pharmacodynamic interaction between the new selective cholesterol absorption inhibitor ezetimibe and simvastatin. British Journal of Clinical Pharmacology. 2002;**54**(3):309-319

[48] Myocardial Infarction Genetics Consortium, I et al. Inactivating mutations in NPC1L1 and protection from coronary heart disease. New England Journal of Medicine. 2014;**371**(22):2072-2082

[49] Ballantyne CM et al. Efficacy and safety of ezetimibe co-administered with simvastatin compared with atorvastatin in adults with hypercholesterolemia. The American Journal of Cardiology. 2004;**93**(12):1487-1494

[50] Morrone D et al. Lipid-altering efficacy of ezetimibe plus statin and statin monotherapy and identification of factors associated with treatment response: A pooled analysis of over 21,000 subjects from 27 clinical trials. Atherosclerosis. 2012;**223**(2):251-261

[51] Cannon CP et al. Ezetimibe added to statin therapy after acute coronary syndromes. The New England Journal of Medicine. 2015;**372**(25):2387-2397

[52] Brar KS. Ezetimibe (Zetia). Medical Journal, Armed Forces India. 2004;**60**(4):388-389

[53] Koshman SL et al. Supratherapeutic response to ezetimibe administered with cyclosporine. Annals of Pharmacotherapy. 2005;**39**(9):1561-1565

[54] Arbel R, Hammerman A, Azuri J. Usefulness of ezetimibe versus evolocumab as add-on therapy for secondary prevention of cardiovascular events in patients with type 2 diabetes mellitus. The American Journal of Cardiology. 2019

Section 4

Adiposity and Non-Tradional Lipid Biomarkers, a Look into the Future

Chapter 9

Adipose Tissue Complexities in Dyslipidemias

Deborah R. Gustafson

Abstract

Adipose tissue is the largest organ in the human body and, in excess, contributes to dyslipidemias and the dysregulation of other vascular and metabolic processes. Adipose tissue is heterogeneous, comprised of several cell types based on morphology, cellular age, and endocrine and paracrine function. Adipose tissue depots are also regional, primarily due to sex differences and genetic variation. Adipose tissue is also characterized as subcutaneous vs. visceral. In addition, fatty deposits exist outside of adipose tissue, such as those surrounding the heart, or as infiltration of skeletal muscle. This review focuses on adipose tissue and its contribution to dyslipidemias. Dyslipidemias are defined as circulating blood lipid levels that are too high or altered. Lipids include both traditional and nontraditional species. Leaving aside traditional definitions, adipose tissue contributes to dyslipidemias in a myriad of ways. To address a small portion of this topic, we reviewed (a) adipose tissue location and cell types, (b) body composition, (c) endocrine adipose, (d) the fat-brain axis, and (e) genetic susceptibility. The influence of these complex aspects of adipose tissue on dyslipidemias and human health, illustrating that, once again, that adipose tissue is a quintessential, multifunctional tissue of the human body, will be summarized.

Keywords: adipose tissue, adipocyte, body weight, body mass index, lipidomics, obesity, leptin, APOE, endocrine, brain

1. Introduction

The World Health Organization (WHO) reports that by 2050, 20% of the world's population will be age 60 years and older [1]. Correspondingly, cardio- and cerebrovascular diseases are the top 10 most common causes of death [2]. Ischemic heart disease is first, followed by stroke (second); Alzheimer's disease (fifth), the disease of the latest life; and type 2 diabetes (T2D, sixth). Vascular diseases comprise four of the top 10 causes of death because of their association with pandemic obesity [2].

Adipose tissue (AT) is the largest organ in the human body. Adiposity (amount of AT) is often classified as overweight and obese using body mass index (BMI, kg/m^2) or Waist Circumference (WC). Over the life course and with aging, BMI is dynamic and evolves in relation to physical growth, puberty, reproductive status, as well as nutritional health and adequacy. The life course evolution of BMI represents an evolutionary metabolism. As such, potential relationships between BMI and accompanying vascular risk factors, such as blood lipid levels, change over the life course and in association with disease. BMI and central adiposity cut points for overweight and obesity as well as for hyperlipidemias (the most common form of

IntechOpen

clinical dyslipidemia) are those associated with mortality and later-life outcomes. See **Tables 1** and **2** for common definitions of these cut points.

Epidemiologic studies exploring the natural history of vascular phenotypes show that levels of body weight, BMI, and blood lipids increase throughout adult life and decline with aging and later-life diseases [3–6]. This is practically illustrated by comparing mid- versus later-life risk scores for late-onset dementia. Obesity and hyperlipidemia are components of mid-life risk scores, but not of later-life risk scores [7–10]. This is often referred to as the "obesity paradox." This contradictory combination of higher disease risk associated with higher mid-life vascular risk and declining vascular phenotypes in the years immediately preceding and at the time of later-onset diseases and death requires further understanding but has very practical implications (**Figure 1**). Lower blood lipid levels and/or rigorous control of blood lipid levels may not be advantageous during the latest life [11]. In addition, genetic

			Disease risk* relative to normal BMI and WC			
	BMI (kg/m^2)	**Obesity class**	**Women ≤88 cm**	**Women >88 cm⁺**	**Men ≤102 cm**	**Men >102 cm⁺**
Underweight	<18.5					
Normal	18.5–24.9					
Overweight	25.0–29.9		Increased	High	Increased	High
Obesity	30.0–34.9	1	High	Very high	High	Very high
	35.0–39.9	2	Very high	Very high	Very high	Very high
Extreme obesity	≥40	3	Extremely high	Extremely high	Extremely high	Extremely high

**Disease risk for T2D, hypertension, and cardiovascular disease.*
⁺Increased Waist Circumference is a marker for increased risk, even in adults of normal weight.

Table 1.
Classification of overweight and obesity by Body Mass Index and Waist Circumference and disease risk based on anthropometric estimates of adipose tissue [108–111].*

mg/dl	**Interpretation**
LDL cholesterol	
<100	Optimal
100–129	Near optimal/above normal
130–159	Borderline high
160–189	High
≥190	Very high
Total cholesterol	
<200	Desirable
200–239	Borderline high
≥240	High
HDL cholesterol	
<40	Low
≥60	High

The National Cholesterol Education Program ATP III Guidelines [112].

Table 2.
Lipid cut points for adults based on blood levels of traditionally measured lipids.

background related to vascular risk such as APOEε4 allele possession, which encodes for a protein on the surface of lipoproteins and influences lipid metabolism and vascular health, has also been associated with late-onset dementia and mortality [12].

The vascular and metabolic complexity and ubiquity of AT demand a more expansive definition of dyslipidemia. Herein the multiple potential contributions of a complex, heterogeneous AT to dyslipidemia phenotypes and human health are described. Dyslipidemias are considered expansively and defined as circulating blood lipid levels that are too high or too low, where lipids refer to more than those listed in **Table 2**. AT contributions to dyslipidemia phenotypes relate to (a) AT location and cell types, (b) body composition, (c) endocrine adipose, (d) the fat-brain axis, and (e) genetic susceptibility (**Figure 2**). This review illustrates that AT is a quintessential, multifunctional tissue of the human body.

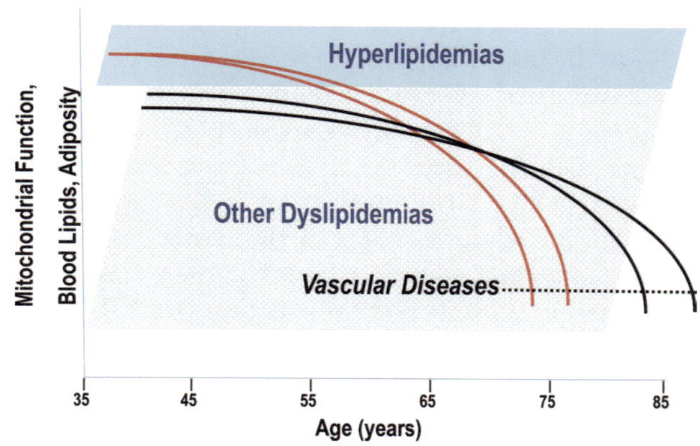

Figure 1.
The biological declines that accompany dyslipidemias.

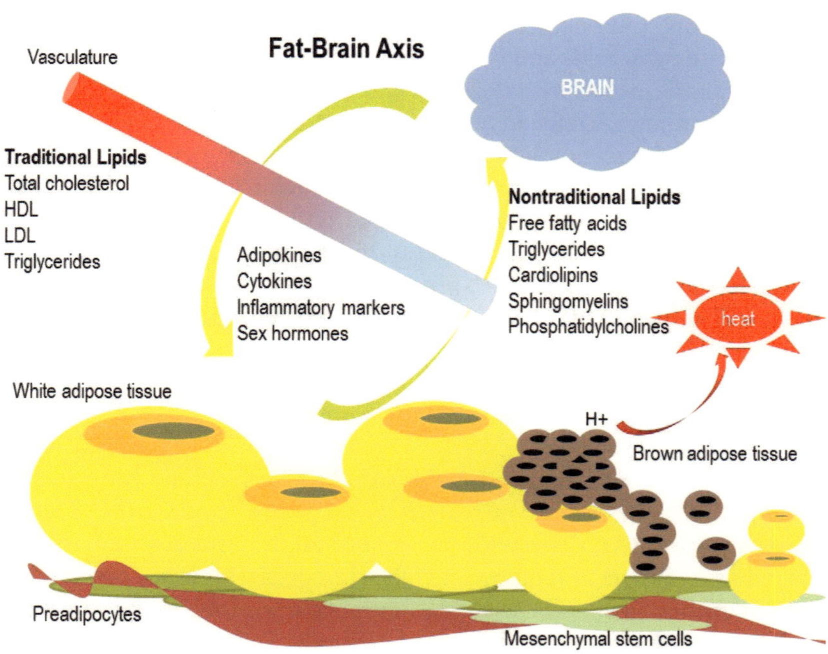

Figure 2.
The heterogeneity of adipose tissue and its dynamic state due to different and evolving cell populations, proportions of WAT/BAT, energetics, and dyslipidemias.

2. Adipose tissue location and cell types

AT consists of multiple cell types exhibiting multiple cellular phenotypes depending on parent cell type and location of deposition [13]. In mammals, body fat compartments include total fat, subcutaneous fat, and internal fat, which is comprised of visceral (within chest, abdomen, and pelvis), nonvisceral (intramuscular, perimuscular), and other fat (e.g., lipomas) [14]. In addition, extra-adipose fatty acid deposits, such as those surrounding the internal organs, including the heart, have profound effects on disease susceptibility and occurrence [15]. Triglyceride deposits in the pancreas have been linked to alterations in insulin secretion; and epicardial fat has been linked to coronary heart disease [15]. While obese levels of BMI are correlated with the amount of these extra-adipose fatty acid deposits, BMI is not a sensitive indicator of their influence on human health and disease, part of which is local alterations in lipid metabolism [15].

AT cells, adipocytes, originate from multipotent mesenchymal stem cell populations (MSCs) in the bone marrow [16]. After initial determination steps, differentiation into a variety of cell types including osteoblasts, myocytes, and chondrocytes may occur [17]. AT-derived stem cells (ADSCs) also differentiate into non-mesenchymal cells (hepatocytes, neurons, pancreatic cells, endothelial cells, and cardiomyocytes) [18]. Characterization of diverse adipocyte populations enhances the understanding of the role of AT in lipid metabolism. Adipocytes differentially secrete hormones and cytokines based on the location of AT or triglyceride deposits; thus location is important for function [19, 20]. The ubiquity of AT and triglyceride deposits throughout the mammalian body and the corresponding autocrine, paracrine, and endocrine effects evidence the importance of the regulatory roles of AT.

AT quality and functionality may be more relevant for vascular and cardiometabolic risk than the total amount of AT [21]. In response to energy surplus, there may be a maladaptive AT expansion in consequent obesity. The significance of this expansion is local and systemic. In response to local excess, hypoxia, dysregulated adipokine secretion, and impaired mitochondrial function may occur. Overtaxed adipocytes release fatty acids and pro-inflammatory factors into the circulation. Subsequent systemic effects include leptin and insulin resistance, altered lipid and glucose metabolism, hypertension, end-organ fat accumulation (e.g., nonalcoholic fatty liver disease), the metabolic syndrome, pro-inflammatory and pro-thrombotic states, and endothelial dysfunction, all of which provide mechanisms for observed associations between obesity and cardio- and cerebrovascular diseases [21, 22]. Specific associations have been observed for dyslipidemias. For example, hypercholesterolemia has been associated with pro-inflammatory macrophage subpopulations in visceral adipose tissue (VAT), while BMI had a prominent effect in white adipose tissue (WAT) only [23].

2.1 White adipose tissue versus brown adipose tissue

There are generally two visual presentations of AT - WAT and brown adipose tissue (BAT) [17, 24]. WAT is characterized by its "white" color, due to a large, lipid-filled cell body. BAT, filled with mitochondria, presents as brown. Several later-onset diseases are characterized by mitochondrial/respiratory chain dysfunction, which emphasizes the potential importance of BAT. Brain and skeletal muscles are the tissues most affected by mitochondrial disorders because they exhibit the highest rates of aerobic metabolism [27, 28]. For example, mitochondria accumulate amyloid-beta, a key protein in Alzheimer's disease [25] that in the brain leads to cellular dysfunction. Brain is comprised of 60% fat [26], yet not AT.

In addition, while not typically containing a large amount of fat, with aging, mitochondria-rich skeletal muscle is infiltrated with extra-AT and triglyceride deposits, leading to a condition called sarcopenia, and contributing to a type of dyslipidemia [29].

WAT and BAT originate from two different stem cell populations in bone marrow. BAT plays an important role, not only in neonatal but in human adult physiology [30].

2.1.1 White adipose tissue

WAT is the predominant AT in mammals. During embryonic development, it arises from lateral plate mesoderm, which forms the underlying stroma or supportive connective tissue. The stroma is highly vascularized and contains progenitor cells that give rise to mature adipocytes. Preadipocytes are immature fat cells that have not yet accumulated lipid. Fully differentiated adipocytes contain lipid in the form of triglyceride when provided with the appropriate nutrients (e.g., glucose) and hormones (e.g., insulin and leptin) [31]. WAT is a storage tissue for fatty acids and other compounds, for example, fat-soluble vitamins [32] and organochlorine pesticides [33].

Not all WAT cells are the same. "Healthy" WAT adipocytes are relatively small and have a high capacity for mitochondrial oxidative phosphorylation, which generates ATP, the cell's aerobic currency. They are also characterized by more efficient cycling of triacylglycerol molecules and fatty acids and de novo lipogenesis. These intrinsic metabolic features of healthy WAT benefit locally and systemically [34].

Unhealthy WAT is attributed to excess or insufficient lipid storage in WAT droplets, which is associated with dyslipidemia, insulin resistance, and increased risk for T2D [35]. WAT adipocyte proteins control adipocyte lipid storage and limit lipid spillover and lipotoxic effects thought to contribute to disease [35]. For example, Caspase-2 is a WAT protein that is associated with abdominal fat accumulation, dyslipidemia, hyperproliferation, and "browning" of adipose [22]. "Overworked" adipocytes are more likely to release fatty acids and pro-inflammatory factors into the circulation that promote organ fat accumulation, insulin resistance, and the metabolic syndrome. Obesity is associated with both hypertrophy and hyperplasia of adipocytes, AT inflammation, impaired extracellular matrix remodeling, fibrosis, and altered secretion of adipokines [36]. These observations illustrate the potential for tissue or regional level dyslipidemias as a result of the changes in the structural, molecular, and metabolic integrity of the adipocyte.

2.1.2 Brown adipose tissue

In contrast to the developmental origins of WAT, mesenchymal stem cells from the paraxial mesoderm give rise to BAT. BAT is identifiable because it expresses the uncoupling protein 1 (UCP1). Myocytes (skeletal muscle cells) are also derived from paraxial mesoderm. Both UCP1-expressing BAT and myocytes express Myf5 (Myf5+) [17], thus further differentiating them from WAT, which are Myf5−. It has been traditionally thought that most BAT disappears fairly quickly with aging; however a significant amount of BAT is present in adults, particularly in paracervical and supraclavicular AT [37], as well as surrounding the kidney and along large blood vessels [38]. At least two types of BAT exist. Myf5+ brown fat is classical brown fat and exists in the aforementioned locations. Myf5− BAT is interspersed in WAT and may sometimes be referred to as "beige" adipose [17, 39].

A notable feature of BAT is an uncoupling of oxidative phosphorylation in response to cold temperatures and other factors that activate the sympathetic nervous system [40]. Free fatty acids are transferred to the mitochondria where they are broken down by two carbon units and undergo β-oxidation. However, UCP1 uncouples oxidation and phosphorylation, leading to futile cycling, adaptive thermogenesis, and the release of energy as heat (instead of ATP) [28].

Using 18F-FDG-PET/CT, it has been observed that women have more BAT mass and activity [41] and that there is proportionately more BAT among older women. However, parallel to later-life body weight and BMI decline, both BAT mass and activity decrease with age, perhaps to a greater extent among men [41]. Seemingly paradoxical, yet as expected, is that amount of BAT is inversely related to BMI during adulthood [42]. Both mass and glucose uptake activity of 18F-FDG-PET/CT-detected BAT decrease with increasing outdoor temperature, age, and BMI [42]. BAT is suggested to be protective for obesity due to its role in adaptive adrenergic thermogenesis [30].

2.1.3 White adipose tissue and brown adipose tissue in aging

Questions that remain are: How are WAT and BAT related to usual aging and aging-related dyslipidemias? How do WAT and BAT relate to observed declines in BMI and blood cholesterol levels with aging? Mitochondrial disorders are common among aging-related diseases [21, 43] and may be exacerbated by BAT. Aging is also associated with a decrease in subcutaneous fat and increase in VAT (located around internal organs). The ratio of BAT to WAT also appears to increase, such that the amount of BAT is inversely correlated with BMI in the elderly [44]. Perhaps there is an evolving proportion of BAT/WAT over the life course that favors anti-obesity and anti-dyslipidemias in mid-life and, among some, accelerated BMI decline in late life, as a result of dysregulated adaptive thermogenesis. There is a paucity of literature linking AT directly to the variety of dyslipidemias that occur with usual aging.

Some data suggest that specific dietary fatty acids are protective for atypical accumulations of body fat, systemic low-grade inflammation, dyslipidemias, and insulin resistance [34]. For example, "healthy adipocytes" are induced in the WAT of obese mice in response to dietary omega-3 polyunsaturated fatty acids (omega-3 PUFAs), especially when combined with other "lifestyle" interventions, for example, moderate calorie restriction. It is unclear whether this relies on the activation of BAT and/or the induction of brite/beige adipocytes in WAT [34].

3. Adipose tissue and body composition

Sex-specific changes in body composition over the life course may lead to profound changes in metabolic feedback loops between the brain and AT, gut, and other peripheral locations. Altered metabolic states may occur as compensatory or to promote or accelerate other aging processes.

With aging, the proportion of fat-to-fat free mass (FFM) increases. Sometimes these changes are accompanied by changes in body weight or BMI, but not necessarily. FFM represents the mass of the organism without fat and is comprised of chemical components, amino acids, water, and minerals. FFM includes the metabolically active mass of cellular elements in the body, which is primarily muscle, organ tissue, and other tissue cells. Resting metabolism occurs in the FFM, which varies by tissue; and FFM depletion occurs in conditions such as cancer, HIV/AIDS, and dementia as well as with age. While there is a decrease in resting metabolic rate (RMR) with decreasing FFM as one ages [45], this decrease does not correspond to changes in body composition nor does it reflect in which body tissues this decrease occurs. It has been hypothesized that a reduction in RMR is due to a combination of decreases in mass and cellular fractions of organs and tissues. It has been shown that increasing age is related to decreasing mass of the brain, kidney, liver, and spleen [46].

4. Endocrine adipose tissue

As aforementioned, AT is measured clinically in several ways. Common clinical and epidemiologic measures include anthropometry, such as BMI, WC, and Waist-to-Hip Ratio (WHR). In addition, are whole and regional body imaging. While the imaging gold standard is Magnetic Resonance Imaging (MRI) or Computed Tomography (CT), Dual X-Ray Absorptiometry (DXA) is also used, as is Bioelectrical Impedance Analysis (BIA). However, given the higher costs of body imaging techniques, peripheral blood-based biomarkers, such as adipokines including leptin, and free fatty acids, measured using lipidomics technologies, are of increasing importance.

Over 600 secretory proteins are attributed to AT [47]. AT is the source of a variety of hormones and cytokines, such as leptin, adiponectin, pro-inflammatory cytokines, and components of complement and the renin-angiotensin system (RAS) [48–50]. A classic example of the endocrine function of AT is its role in female reproductive health. Hypotheses related to a critical percentage of body adiposity for the initiation of menarche in females, such as the Frisch hypothesis, were first reported in 1973 [51]. In addition, AT is the primary source of bioactive estrogen (as estrone, E1) in postmenopausal women via aromatase [52]. AT-derived sex hormones also link adiposity and changes in adiposity to the occurrence of dyslipidemias. For example, aromatase knockout mice exhibit elevated circulating levels of leptin and cholesterol concomitant with lower estrogen levels than wild-type controls [53]. The metabolic implications of AT are wide ranging, and knowledge related to this phenomenon is far from complete.

Changes in body composition over the adult life and corresponding influences on dyslipidemias are not yet fully characterized. Declines in both BMI and blood cholesterol levels [3, 54] occur with aging; however there is a relative lack of published studies on changes over time, across populations and with lipid-lowering treatments. One may speculate that the changes in adiposity observed in aging correspond directly to changes in blood levels of AT metabolites, including FFA, and traditionally measured lipids [33]. There may be important temporal, acute changes occurring that are not easily understood when using cross-sectional analyses depending on chronological and biological age. The complexity of AT endocrinology and related systems is well-illustrated by the range of medications used for vascular diseases of old age. Several of these medications differentially influence body weight [11, 55] and subsequent blood lipid levels. In addition, studies of adults with cerebral small vessel disease or HIV-related adiposity syndromes allow continued evaluation of the aforementioned, co-occurring factors and partitioning out of different adiposity pathways [49, 56, 57]. AT contributions to dyslipidemias may be apparent across any body weight or BMI, with or without the use of lipid-lowering agents.

Hormones and cytokines produced by AT such as leptin and adiponectin are involved in the regulation and dysregulation of nutrient utilization, as well as inflammation, endothelial dysfunction, hypertension, and atherogenesis [58]. In addition, combinations of hormones, such as insulin and leptin, interact in various processes such as nutrient utilization to augment effects. Two AT hormones, leptin and adiponectin, are described here as well as a discussion of lipidomics approaches. **Table 3** contains several selected examples of adipokines that may be associated with dyslipidemias.

4.1 Leptin

Leptin is a 16 kDa protein hormone discovered in 1994. While deemed to be the putative obesity hormone in the mid-1990s [59], with effects possibly mediated by an impaired BBB [60], it did not become the answer to the current obesity epidemic as originally hoped. The amount of AT is positively related to blood leptin levels, as AT is the major source of this hormone [61, 62]. The Prospective Study of Women in Gothenburg, Sweden, shows mid-life correlations of r = 0.67 and late-life correlations of r = 0.61 between BMI and blood leptin levels [6]. Similar BMI-leptin correlations are also observed in "at-risk" populations such as women with HIV infection and cerebral small vessel disease (unpublished observations).

Adipose tissue secretory product	Function
Adiponectin	Insulin sensitizer; circulating levels inversely correlated to dyslipidemias, insulin resistance, metabolic syndrome, obesity, T2D, and cardiovascular diseases [49, 50, 113]
Chemerin	Regulates adipogenesis and mature adipocyte metabolism; elevated in obesity, dyslipidemia, T2D, and osteoporosis; a marker of inflammation and metabolic syndrome [114]
Hepatocyte growth factor (HGF)	Angiogenic and mitogenic effects; linked to vascular diseases; elevated in obese adults and adolescents [115, 116]
Interleukin (IL)-6	Pro-inflammatory, upregulated in obesity, can exacerbate CVD and metabolic syndrome [113]
Leptin	Regulates body weight via decreasing appetite and increasing sympathetic nervous activity [49, 50, 117, 118]
Neuregulin 4	Regulates energy metabolism; associated with BMI, WHR, triglycerides, and other metabolites; secreted from brown/beige AT [119–121]
Nerve growth factor (NGF)	Correlated with waist-to-hip ratio (WHR); associated with NGF and leptin, T2D, cardiovascular disease, and stroke [122]
Omentin-1	Associated with VAT, dyslipidemia, metabolic syndrome, T2D, and cardiovascular disease; inhibits the inflammatory response and improves insulin resistance; vasodilatory [123]
Plasminogen activator inhibitor-1 (PAI-1)	Associated with central obesity; mediates fibrinolysis; crosses an intact blood-brain barrier [124, 125]
Progranulin	Higher in obesity, insulin resistance, T2D, fatty liver disease; associated with inflammation, growth-promotion, and neuroprotection [126]
Resistin	Pro-inflammatory; produced in response to pro-inflammatory cytokines [113, 127]
Retinol-binding protein (RBP)	Elevated in obesity; implicated in insulin resistance; associated with triglyceride and small HDL levels [128, 129]
Tumor necrosis factor (TNF)-α	Pro-inflammatory; upregulated in obesity; exacerbates cardiovascular disease and metabolic syndrome [113]

Table 3.
Examples of adipose tissue secretory products and their functions that may be disrupted in dyslipidemias.

Classical functions of leptin include signaling inadequate energy stores through the regulation of food intake, regulation of energy expenditure, improving insulin sensitivity, facilitating lipolysis, inhibiting lipogenesis, and reducing intracellular lipids [63]. In addition, leptin plays a permissive role in neuroendocrine immune function [63]. In obesity, there occurs a phenomenon called "leptin resistance." Analogous to insulin resistance, leptin resistance implies decreased tissue sensitivity to leptin, which leads to dyslipidemia [64]. In contrast, leptin replacement therapy (metreleptin) is used to treat lipodystrophy syndromes characterized by a loss of AT that also leads to dyslipidemia [65].

Understanding interactions between leptin and insulin in the brain may weave together the interrelationship of adiposity and T2D. T2D is also associated with dyslipidemias. Not only leptin, as aforementioned, but insulin interacts directly with hypothalamic nuclei, and it appears that both are involved in the manifestation of insulin resistance. The pro-opiomelanocortin (POMC) neurons in the hypothalamus express both leptin and insulin receptors and regulate energy balance and glucose homeostasis. Experimental mouse models lacking both leptin and insulin receptors in POMC neurons display systemic insulin resistance, which is distinct from what occurs with the single deletion of either receptor. These mice also show alterations in sex hormone levels that reduce fertility. Thus, direct actions of both insulin and leptin on POMC neurons appear to be required to maintain normal glucose homeostasis and reproductive function [66] and will therefore influence blood lipid levels and AT-related FFA metabolism. It has also been proposed that cross talk between leptin and insulin occurs within a network of cells rather than within individual POMC neurons [67].

In relation to AT, it has been shown in mouse models that leptin regulates body weight via decreasing appetite and increasing sympathetic nervous activity. This, in turn, increases energy expenditure in interscapular BAT [68], and correspondingly there is an increase in BAT temperature. Neurons in the dorsomedial hypothalamus appear to mediate this thermogenic response to hyperleptinemia in obese mice, and a functional melanocortin system is not required. Because the sympathetic nervous system contributes in regulating blood pressure, heart rate, and hepatic glucose production, selective leptin resistance may be a crucial mechanism linking adiposity, BAT, and dyslipidemias [64, 69].

4.2 Adiponectin

Adiponectin (also known as ACRP30) is an effective insulin sensitizer; circulating levels are inversely correlated to dyslipidemias, insulin resistance, metabolic syndrome, obesity, T2D, and cardiovascular diseases. These observations, as for leptin, appear consistent cross-culturally. Adiponectin exists as complex multimeric isoforms comprised of high molecular weight (HMW), hexamers, and trimers [70]. HMW adiponectin or HMW adiponectin/total adiponectin may be better indicators of insulin sensitivity than total adiponectin in obesity, T2D, and cardiovascular disease [70]. Adiponectin is produced not only by AT but by numerous other tissues including the brain. BMI is inversely related to circulating adiponectin. The Prospective Study of Women in Gothenburg, Sweden, shows late-life correlations of $r = -0.29$, between BMI and blood adiponectin levels (unpublished). Similar correlations are observed in women with HIV infection and in adults with cerebral small vessel disease (unpublished observations). In addition, since adiponectin is a VAT marker and only moderately correlated with BMI, it may not be associated in a similar fashion with lipid metabolism when compared to BMI or other anthropometric measures [71]. Interestingly, the adiponectin/leptin ratio has been proposed as a better indicator of AT dysfunction and cardiometabolic risk [72].

4.3 Lipidomics

Lipidomics platforms comprised of mass spectrometry/gas chromatography are used to discriminate among levels of obesity and to identify dyslipidemias characterized by nontraditional lipid biomarkers. These alternative lipid species may be associated with obesity-related chronic diseases as well as for accumulation of excess AT [73–75]. For example, obesity, independent of genetic influences, has been related to [1] increases in lysophosphatidylcholines and lipids observed in pro-inflammatory and pro-atherogenic conditions and [2] decreases in other phospholipids, which are known to have antioxidant properties [76]. Certain conditions characterized by lipodystrophies and/or higher levels of AT, such as HIV infection, facilitate studies of traditionally and nontraditionally defined dyslipidemias and altered energy metabolism [77–79]. Nontraditional blood lipids of importance may include cardiolipins, sphingomyelins, phosphatidylcholines, and nonesterified fatty acids [80]. While the differential bioactivities of these lipids are unknown, mitochondrial dysfunction may underlie some of these differences among disease states and between diseased and healthy states [81, 82].

Cardiolipins (CLs) are an example of a class of lipids that may be informative for obesity, dyslipidemias, and associated diseases. CLs are diphosphatidylglycerol molecules with four acyl groups that can bind four fatty acids. In human circulation, these are usually 18-carbon fatty acids [80% linoleic acid (18:2(n−6))] [83]. CLs in the central nervous system contain a wider range of fatty acids including palmitic, stearic (18:0), oleic (18:1), arachidonic (20:0), and docosahexaenoic acids (22:6) (over 100 molecular species); and lymphoblast CLs contain only monoenoic fatty acids. CLs are predominant in the heart (where first discovered), liver, and brain [83]. Individuals with obesity, T2D, or heart failure have elevated levels of serum free fatty acids [84] that promote lipotoxicity of cardiomyocytes [85]; and profound changes in CLs' composition occur in T2D. Since the brain is approximately 60% fat [26] and obesity is associated with later-onset cognitive impairments and dementias [50, 55, 86], perhaps the abundance of these circulating lipid species is of multisystem pathological significance. This multisystem role of CL alterations contributing to mitochondrial dysfunction in particular makes them especially interesting [87].

CLs are mitochondrial membrane phospholipids present mostly in the inner membrane, where they comprise ~20% of the total lipid content [88]. However, CLs are also transferred to the outer mitochondrial membrane and can comprise ~25% of the lipid content at locations where fission and fusion occur. Inner membrane CLs, the site of the electron transport chain, and the electrochemical gradient involved in ATP production [89] are evidence of the likely role of CLs in mitochondrial bioenergetics. CLs are required for optimal functioning of several inner mitochondrial membrane proteins and enzymes [89–94], including those involved in electron transport chain-mediated oxidative phosphorylation and coupled respiration [95]. CLs appear to be an integral component of these proteins and critical for folding, structure, and function. CLs are prone to reactive oxygen species-induced oxidative damage and important during mitochondrial apoptosis [88]. CL oxidation is observed in insulin resistance [96], obesity [97], and nonalcoholic fatty liver disease [98]. Metabolic dysfunction pertaining to CLs in brain mitochondria is suggested in neurodegenerative diseases, including Alzheimer's disease and Parkinson's disease [99]. In Parkinson's disease, for example, α-synuclein seems to form an oligomer that binds to mitochondrial membrane CLs, thereby disrupting integrity and impairing function [100, 101].

5. The fat-brain axis

Mechanisms whereby AT and its secretory products affect peripheral lipid metabolism are centrally coordinated [102]. For example, leptin and adiponectin, peripheral AT signals, interact with hypothalamic nuclei such as the arcuate nucleus. These interactions trigger the release of orexigenic and anorectic peptides from PMC neurons. These peptides exert peripheral effects, modulating food intake, reproduction, water balance, body temperature, and energy balance. In addition, leptin and adiponectin have been shown to enhance synaptic plasticity. This is illustrated in studies of Alzheimer neuropathology, where amyloid is deposited in the areas of the hypothalamus such as the arcuate nucleus, where it potentially interferes with usual physiologic influences of AT and its primary hormones, such as leptin and adiponectin as well as downstream events and feedback loops [49, 50]. The influence of Alzheimer pathology on areas of the brain involved in homeostatic regulation may explain the decline in levels of blood cholesterol and body weight observed in prodromal and overt dementia [11]. In addition, data show that leptin exerts control over hepatic lipid metabolism via the central nervous system and via peripheral nerves. Central regulation of lipid metabolism in WAT and BAT may also contribute to hepatic lipid content indirectly via FFA release and changes in lipoprotein clearance. Impairments in these pathways may contribute to dyslipidemias [102].

6. Genes related to adipose tissue

Given published associations of adiposity with brain outcomes including Alzheimer's Disease (AD) [refs 1, 5, 6, 11, 48–50, 55, 56, 57, 103, 104], understanding the potential role of adiposity- and lipid-related susceptibility genes in AD may provide insights regarding biological underpinnings related to AT. Genes related to AD susceptibility may have a modifying effect on the relationship between AT, dyslipidemias, and aging. Several genes have been identified that link AT and corresponding vascular risk to cognitive decline, AD susceptibility, and pathological processes. APOE and FTO are two of them.

The APOE gene encodes for a protein on the surface of lipoproteins that aids in lipoprotein metabolism [12]. The APOEε4 allele is a known susceptibility allele for dementia. It also modifies the association between BMI decline, often observed to a great extent among those developing dementia [55], dementia [103], as well as dementia progression [104].

FTO ("fatso") is an obesity-susceptibility gene and related to T2D. The resulting protein product of FTO appears to be a member of the non-heme dioxygenase (Fe(II)- and 2-oxoglutarate-dependent dioxygenases) superfamily. FTO mRNA is the most abundant in the brain, particularly in hypothalamic nuclei governing energy balance. Levels in the arcuate nucleus are regulated by feeding and fasting [105], thus potentially integrating AT hormones in the fat-brain axis. The influence of lipid type is also modulated by FTO [106].

The existence of susceptibility genes such as APOE and FTO points to the potential role of developmental origins in the life course trajectories of lipids and anthropometric measures of AT, such as BMI, in relation to brain structure and function as well as age- and lipid-related diseases of the brain [107]. Genetic susceptibility and gene-environment interactions, especially over the life course, remain largely unexplored. Stratification of population samples on the basis of these important genotypes lends insight into innate susceptibility-related AT over the life course [103].

7. In conclusion: adipose, a quintessential multifunctional tissue

Understanding the complexity of AT and its role in dyslipidemia in the periphery and its interactions with the brain is paramount to the development of intervention strategies focused on obesity-related exposures, correlates, and outcomes. Issues related to the epidemiology, adipocyte subpopulations, differential energetics, endocrinology, amyloid, and genetics are aspects of adiposity requiring further investigation.

Based on this review, several suggestions can be made for future research. The use of simple anthropometric indicators in epidemiologic studies is somewhat obsolete, particularly for elderly populations. Anthropometric indicators could be replaced by measures reflecting potential biological functions and structures of AT. These measures include traditional and nontraditional lipid species as well as endocrine metabolites of AT that are measureable in peripheral fluids. Whole body imaging is also important. Improving measures of adipocyte subpopulations accompanied by improved methods for biopsying and measuring these important cells and/or their activities in epidemiologic and clinical studies are needed. As adipocytes are produced throughout the life span of mammals, and in response to the changing status of the organism, they may prove to be important gauges and influencers of metabolic health, not only peripherally but centrally for the brain. Therefore, brain imaging measures may be useful as preclinical indicators of susceptibility as well as comprising outcomes associated with the adiposity exposure. Enriching future studies for certain genetic or "at-risk" subgroups may lend additional insights. In time, our appreciation for AT and its complexity will only grow and mature to ultimately improve human health.

Acknowledgements

This review was supported in part by funding from the State University of New York and the National Institutes of Health/National Heart Lung and Blood Institute U01HL146202.

Conflict of interest

The author declares no conflict of interest.

Author details

Deborah R. Gustafson[1,2]

1 Department of Neurology, State University of New York Downstate Medical Center, New York, USA

2 Department of Health and Education, University of Skövde, Skövde, Sweden

*Address all correspondence to: deborah.gustafson@downstate.edu

References

[1] World Health Organization. Health in Older Age. Geneva: World Health Organization; 2015

[2] World Health Organization. Top Ten Causes of Death. Report No.: Contract No.: Fact Sheet No 310. World Health Organization, 2017

[3] Mielke MM, Zandi PP, Shao H, Waern M, Ostling S, Guo X, et al. The 32-year relationship between cholesterol and dementia from midlife to late life. Neurology. 2010;**75**(21):1888-1895

[4] Solomon A, Kareholt I, Ngandu T, Winblad B, Nissinen A, Tuomilehto J, et al. Serum cholesterol changes after midlife and late-life cognition: Twenty-one-year follow-up study. Neurology. 2007;**68**(10):751-756

[5] Stewart R, Masaki K, Xue QL, Peila R, Petrovitch H, White LR, et al. A 32-year prospective study of change in body weight and incident dementia: The Honolulu-Asia Aging Study. Archives of Neurology. 2005;**62**(1):55-60

[6] Gustafson DR, Backman K, Joas E, Waern M, Ostling S, Guo X, et al. 37 years of body mass index and dementia: Observations from the prospective population study of women in Gothenburg, Sweden. Journal of Alzheimer's Disease: JAD. 2012;**28**(1):163-171

[7] Exalto LG, Quesenberry CP, Barnes D, Kivipelto M, Biessels GJ, Whitmer RA. Midlife risk score for the prediction of dementia four decades later. Alzheimer's & Dementia. 2014;**10**(5):562-570

[8] Kivipelto M, Ngandu T, Laatikainen T, Winblad B, Soininen H, Tuomilehto J. Risk score for the prediction of dementia risk in 20 years among middle aged people: A longitudinal, population-based study. Lancet Neurology. 2006;**5**(9):735-741

[9] Barnes DE, Beiser AS, Lee A, Langa KM, Koyama A, Preis SR, et al. Development and validation of a brief dementia screening indicator for primary care. Alzheimer's & Dementia. 2014;**10**(6):656-665

[10] Walters K, Hardoon S, Petersen I, Iliffe S, Omar RZ, Nazareth I, et al. Predicting dementia risk in primary care: Development and validation of the Dementia Risk Score using routinely collected data. BMC Medicine. 2016;**14**:6

[11] Gustafson DR. Epidemiology informs clinical trials of cognitive impairments and late-onset dementias. Journal of Neurology & Neuromedicine. 2018;**3**:13-18

[12] Guerreiro RJ, Gustafson DR, Hardy J. The genetic architecture of Alzheimer's disease: Beyond APP. PSENs and APOE. Neurobiology of Aging. 2012;**33**(3):437-456

[13] Prunet-Marcassus B, Cousin B, Caton D, Andre M, Penicaud L, Casteilla L. From heterogeneity to plasticity in adipose tissues: Site-specific differences. Experimental Cell Research. 2006;**312**(6):727-736

[14] Shen W, Wang Z, Punyanita M, Lei J, Sinav A, Kral JG, et al. Adipose tissue quantification by imaging methods: A proposed classification. Obesity Research. 2003;**11**(1):5-16

[15] McGavock JM, Victor RG, Unger RH, Szczepaniak LS. Adiposity of the heart, revisited. Annals of Internal Medicine. 2006;**144**:517-524

[16] Kawai M, Devlin MJ, Rosen CJ. Fat targets for skeletal health. Nature Reviews Rheumatology. 2009;**5**(7):365-372

[17] Enerback S. Brown adipose tissue in humans. International Journal of Obesity. 2010;**34**(Suppl 1):S43-S46

[18] Yarak S, Okamoto OK. Human adipose-derived stem cells: Current challenges and clinical perspectives. Anais Brasileiros de Dermatologia. 2010;**85**(5):647-656

[19] Ofori EK, Conde Alonso S, Correas-Gomez L, Carnero EA, Zwygart K, Hugues H, et al. Thigh and abdominal adipose tissue depot associations with testosterone levels in postmenopausal females. Clinical Endocrinology. 2019;**90**(3):433-439

[20] Ma X, Lee P, Chisholm DJ, James DE. Control of adipocyte differentiation in different fat depots; implications for pathophysiology or therapy. Frontiers in Endocrinology. 2015;**6**(1):1-8. DOI: 10.3389/fendo.2015.00001

[21] Koliaki C, Liatis S, Kokkinos A. Obesity and cardiovascular disease: Revisiting an old relationship. Metabolism. 2019;**92**:98-107

[22] Machado MV, Michelotti GA, Jewell ML, Pereira TA, Xie G, Premont RT, et al. Caspase-2 promotes obesity, the metabolic syndrome and nonalcoholic fatty liver disease. Cell Death & Disease. 2016;7:e2096

[23] Kralova Lesna I, Petras M, Cejkova S, Kralova A, Fronek J, Janousek L, et al. Cardiovascular disease predictors and adipose tissue macrophage polarization: Is there a link? European Journal of Preventive Cardiology. 2018;**25**(3):328-334

[24] Ravussin E, Galgani JE. The implication of brown adipose tissue for humans. Annual Review of Nutrition. 2011;**31**:33-47

[25] Manczak M, Anekonda TS, Henson E, Park BS, Quinn J, Reddy PH. Mitochondria are a direct site of A beta accumulation in Alzheimer's disease neurons: Implications for free radical generation and oxidative damage in disease progression. Human Molecular Genetics. 2006;**15**(9):1437-1449

[26] Chang CY, Ke DS, Chen JY. Essential fatty acids and human brain. Acta Neurologica Taiwanica. 2009;**18**(4):231-241

[27] Lecoultre V, Ravussin E. Brown adipose tissue and aging. Current Opinion in Clinical Nutrition and Metabolic Care. 2011;**14**(1):1-6

[28] Rousset S, Alves-Guerra MC, Mozo J, Miroux B, Cassard-Doulcier AM, Bouillaud F, et al. The biology of mitochondrial uncoupling proteins. Diabetes. 2004;**53**(Suppl 1):S130-S135

[29] Huffman DM, Barzilai N. Contribution of adipose tissue to health span and longevity. Interdisciplinary Topics in Gerontology. 2010;**37**:1-19

[30] Nedergaard J, Cannon B. Brown adipose tissue as a heat-producing thermoeffector. Handbook of Clinical Neurology. 2018;**156**:137-152

[31] UNAIDS Report on the Global AIDS Epidemic. Joint United Nations Programme on HIV/AIDS (UNAIDS), 2010 Contract No.: UNAIDS/10.11E | JC1958E

[32] Kohlmeier L, Kohlmeier M. Adipose tissue as a medium for epidemiologic exposure assessment. Environmental Health Perspectives. 1995;**103**(Suppl 3):99-106

[33] Lee DH, Porta M, Lind L, Lind PM, Jacobs DR Jr. Neurotoxic chemicals in adipose tissue: A role in puzzling findings on obesity and dementia. Neurology. 2018;**90**(4):176-182

[34] Kuda O, Rossmeisl M, Kopecky J. Omega-3 fatty acids and adipose tissue biology. Molecular Aspects of Medicine. 2018;**64**:147-160

[35] Konige M, Wang H, Sztalryd C. Role of adipose specific lipid droplet proteins in maintaining whole body energy homeostasis. Biochimica et Biophysica Acta. 2014;**1842**(3):393-401

[36] Rodriguez A, Ezquerro S, Mendez-Gimenez L, Becerril S, Fruhbeck G. Revisiting the adipocyte: A model for integration of cytokine signaling in the regulation of energy metabolism. American Journal of Physiology Endocrinology and Metabolism. 2015;**309**(8):E691-E714

[37] Virtanen KA, Lidell ME, Orava J, Heglind M, Westergren R, Niemi T, et al. Functional brown adipose tissue in healthy adults. The New England Journal of Medicine. 2009;**360**(15):1518-1525

[38] Seale P, Bjork B, Yang W, Kajimura S, Chin S, Kuang S, et al. PRDM16 controls a brown fat/skeletal muscle switch. Nature. 2008;**454**(7207):961-967

[39] Mattson MP. Perspective: Does brown fat protect against diseases of aging? Ageing Research Reviews. 2010;**9**(1):69-76

[40] Ducharme NA, Bickel PE. Lipid droplets in lipogenesis and lipolysis. Endocrinology. 2008;**149**(3):942-949

[41] Pfannenberg C, Werner MK, Ripkens S, Stef I, Deckert A, Schmadl M, et al. Impact of age on the relationships of brown adipose tissue with sex and adiposity in humans. Diabetes. 2010;**59**(7):1789-1793

[42] Ouellet V, Routhier-Labadie A, Bellemare W, Lakhal-Chaieb L, Turcotte E, Carpentier AC, et al. Outdoor temperature, age, sex, body mass index, and diabetic status determine the prevalence, mass, and glucose-uptake activity of 18F-FDG-detected BAT in humans. The Journal of Clinical Endocrinology and Metabolism. 2011;**96**(1):192-199

[43] Barnes PJ. Mechanisms of development of multimorbidity in the elderly. The European Respiratory Journal. 2015;**45**(3):790-806

[44] Cypess AM, Lehman S, Williams G, Tal I, Rodman D, Goldfine AB, et al. Identification and importance of brown adipose tissue in adult humans. The New England Journal of Medicine. 2009;**360**(15):1509-1517

[45] Chapman IM. Obesity paradox during aging. Interdisciplinary Topics in Gerontology. 2010;**37**:20-36

[46] St-Onge MP, Gallagher D. Body composition changes with aging: The cause or the result of alterations in metabolic rate and macronutrient oxidation? Nutrition. 2010;**26**(2):152-155

[47] Lehr S, Hartwig S, Sell H. Adipokines: A treasure trove for the discovery of biomarkers for metabolic disorders. Proteomics Clinical applications. 2012;**6**(1-2):91-101

[48] Gustafson D. A life course of adiposity and dementia. European Journal of Pharmacology. 2008;**585**(1):163-175

[49] Arnoldussen IA, Kiliaan AJ, Gustafson DR. Obesity and dementia: Adipokines interact with the brain. European Neuropsychopharmacology. 2014;**24**(12):1982-1999

[50] Kiliaan AJ, Arnoldussen IA, Gustafson DR. Adipokines: A link between obesity and dementia? The Lancet Neurology. 2014;**13**(9):913-923

[51] Frisch RE, Revelle R, Cook S. Components of weight at menarche and the initiation of the adolescent growth spurt in girls: Estimated total water, llean body weight and fat. Human Biology. 1973;**45**(3):469-483

[52] Campbell (nee Gustafson) DR, Kurzer MS. Flavonoid inhibition of aromatase enzyme activity in human preadipocytes. The Journal of Steroid Biochemistry and Molecular Biology. 1993;**46**(3):381-388

[53] Jones ME, Thorburn AW, Britt KL, Hewitt KN, Wreford NG, Proietto J, et al. Aromatase-deficient (ArKO) mice have a phenotype of increased adiposity. Proceedings of the National Academy of Sciences of the United States of America. 2000;**97**(23):12735-12740

[54] Stewart R, White LR, Xue QL, Launer LJ. Twenty-six-year change in total cholesterol levels and incident dementia: The Honolulu-Asia Aging Study. Archives of Neurology. 2007;(64):103-107

[55] Franx BAA, Arnoldussen IAC, Kiliaan AJ, Gustafson DR. Weight loss in patients with dementia: Considering the potential impact of pharmacotherapy. Drugs & Aging. 2017;**34**(6):425-436

[56] Gustafson DR, Mielke MM, Keating SA, Holman S, Minkoff H, Crystal HA. Leptin, adiponectin and cognition in middle-aged HIV-infected and uninfected women. The Brooklyn Women's Interagency HIV Study. Journal of Gerontology and Geriatric Research. 2015;**4**(5):240. DOI: 10.4172/2167-7182.1000240

[57] Arnoldussen IAC, Gustafson DR-f, van Lejsen EMC, de Leeuw FE, Kiliaan AJ. Adiposity is related to cerebrovascular and brain volumetry outcomes in the RUN DMC study. Neurology. In press

[58] Duvnjak L, Duvnjak M. The metabolic syndrome—An ongoing story. Journal of Physiology and Pharmacology. 2009;**60**(Suppl 7):19-24

[59] Maffei M, Halaas J, Ravussin E, Pratley RE, Lee GH, Zhang Y, et al. Leptin levels in human and rodent: Measurement of plasma leptin and ob RNA in obese and weight-reduced subjects. Nature Medicine. 1995;**1**(11):1155-1161

[60] Banks W. Is obesity a disease of the blood-brain barrier? Physiological, pathological, and evolutionary considerations. Current Pharmaceutical Design. 2003;**9**:801-809

[61] Friedman J, Halaas L. Leptin and the regulation of body weight in mammals. Nature. 1998;**22**:763-770

[62] Lissner L, Karlsson C, Lindroos AK, Sjostrom L, Carlsson B, Carlsson L, et al. Birth weight, adulthood BMI, and subsequent weight gain in relation to leptin levels in Swedish women. Obesity Research. 1999;**7**(2):150-154

[63] Bluher S, Mantzoros CS. Leptin in humans: Lessons from translational research. The American Journal of Clinical Nutrition. 2009;**89**(3):991S-997S

[64] Gruzdeva O, Borodkina D, Uchasova E, Dyleva Y, Barbarash O. Leptin resistance: Underlying mechanisms and diagnosis. Diabetes, Metabolic Syndrome and Obesity. 2019;**12**:191-198

[65] Araujo-Vilar D, Santini F. Diagnosis and treatment of lipodystrophy: A step-by-step approach. Journal of Endocrinological Investigation. 2019;**42**(1):61-73

[66] Hill JW, Elias CF, Fukuda M, Williams KW, Berglund ED, Holland WL, et al. Direct insulin and leptin action on pro-opiomelanocortin neurons is required for normal glucose homeostasis and fertility. Cell Metabolism. 2010;**11**(4):286-297

[67] Williams KW, Margatho LO, Lee CE, Choi M, Lee S, Scott MM, et al. Segregation of acute leptin and insulin effects in distinct populations of arcuate proopiomelanocortin neurons. The Journal of Neuroscience. 2010;**30**(7):2472-2479

[68] Enriori PJ, Sinnayah P, Simonds SE, Garcia Rudaz C, Cowley MA. Leptin action in the dorsomedial hypothalamus

increases sympathetic tone to brown adipose tissue in spite of systemic leptin resistance. The Journal of Neuroscience: The Official Journal of the Society for Neuroscience. 2011;**31**(34):12189-12197

[69] Kanoski SE, Hayes MR, Greenwald HS, Fortin SM, Gianessi CA, Gilbert JR, et al. Hippocampal leptin signaling reduces food intake and modulates food-related memory processing. Neuropsychopharmacology: Official Publication of the American College of Neuropsychopharmacology. 2011;**36**(9):1859-1870

[70] Sinha MK, Songer T, Xiao Q, Sloan JH, Wang J, Ji S, et al. Analytical validation and biological evaluation of a high molecular-weight adiponectin ELISA. Clinical Chemistry. 2007;**53**(12):2144-2151

[71] Drolet EA. Fat depot-specific impact of visceral obesity on adipocyte adiponectin release in women. Obesity (Silver Spring). 2008;**17**:424-430

[72] Fruhbeck G, Catalan V, Rodriguez A, Gomez-Ambrosi J. Adiponectin-leptin ratio: A promising index to estimate adipose tissue dysfunction. Relation with obesity-associated cardiometabolic risk. Adipocytes. 2018;**7**(1):57-62

[73] Meikle PJ, Wong G, Barlow CK, Kingwell BA. Lipidomics: Potential role in risk prediction and therapeutic monitoring for diabetes and cardiovascular disease. Pharmacology & Therapeutics. 2014;**143**(1):12-23

[74] Tonks KT, Coster AC, Christopher MJ, Chaudhuri R, Xu A, Gagnon-Bartsch J, et al. Skeletal muscle and plasma lipidomic signatures of insulin resistance and overweight/obesity in humans. Obesity (Silver Spring). 2016;**24**(4):908-916

[75] Alshehry ZH, Mundra PA, Barlow CK, Mellett NA, Wong G, McConville MJ, et al. Plasma lipidomic profiles improve on traditional risk factors for the prediction of cardiovascular events in type 2 diabetes mellitus. Circulation. 2016;**134**(21):1637-1650

[76] Pietilainen KH, Sysi-Aho M, Rissanen A, Seppanen-Laakso T, Yki-Jarvinen H, Kaprio J, et al. Acquired obesity is associated with changes in the serum lipidomic profile independent of genetic effects—A monozygotic twin study. PLoS One. 2007;**2**(2):e218

[77] Fitch KV, Guggina LM, Keough HM, Dolan Looby SE, Hadigan C, Anderson EJ, et al. Decreased respiratory quotient in relation to resting energy expenditure in HIV-infected and noninfected subjects. Metabolism. 2009;**58**(5):608-615

[78] Mittelsteadt AL, Hileman CO, Harris SR, Payne KM, Gripshover BM, McComsey GA. Effects of HIV and antiretroviral therapy on resting energy expenditure in adult HIV-infected women—A matched, prospective, cross-sectional study. Journal of the Academy of Nutrition and Dietetics. 2013;**113**(8):1037-1043

[79] Vassimon HS, de Paula FJ, Machado AA, Monteiro JP, Jordao AA Jr. Hypermetabolism and altered substrate oxidation in HIV-infected patients with lipodystrophy. Nutrition. 2012;**28**(9):912-916

[80] Rauschert S, Uhl O, Koletzko B, Kirchberg F, Mori TA, Huang RC, et al. Lipidomics reveals associations of phospholipids with obesity and insulin resistance in young adults. The Journal of Clinical Endocrinology and Metabolism. 2016;**101**(3):871-879

[81] Brown T, Confrancesco J Jr. Update from the 6th international workshop on adverse drug reactions and lipodystrophy in HIV. The Hopkins HIV Report. 2005;**17**(1):4-5 8

[82] Willig AL, Kramer PA, Chacko BK, Darley-Usmar VM, Heath SL,

Overton ET. Monocyte bioenergetic function is associated with body composition in virologically suppressed HIV-infected women. Redox Biology. 2017;**12**:648-656

[83] Paradies G, Paradies V, Ruggiero FM, Petrosillo G. Cardiolipin and mitochondrial function in health and disease. Antioxidants & Redox Signaling. 2014;**20**(12):1925-1953

[84] Mantena SK, King AL, Andringa KK, Eccleston HB, Bailey SM. Mitochondrial dysfunction and oxidative stress in the pathogenesis of alcohol- and obesity-induced fatty liver diseases. Free Radical Biology & Medicine. 2008;**44**(7):1259-1272

[85] Rolo AP, Teodoro JS, Palmeira CM. Role of oxidative stress in the pathogenesis of nonalcoholic steatohepatitis. Free Radical Biology & Medicine. 2012;**52**(1):59-69

[86] Gustafson D. BMI and dementia: Feast or famine for the brain? The Lancet Diabetes and Endocrinology. 2015;**3**(6):397-398

[87] Paradies G, Paradies V, Ruggiero FM, Petrosillo G. Oxidative stress, cardiolipin and mitochondrial dysfunction in nonalcoholic fatty liver disease. World Journal of Gastroenterology. 2014;**20**(39):14205-14218

[88] Frohman MA. Role of mitochondrial lipids in guiding fission and fusion. Journal of Molecular Medicine (Berlin, Germany). 2015;**93**(3):263-269

[89] Schlame M, Rua D, Greenberg ML. The biosynthesis and functional role of cardiolipin. Progress in Lipid Research. 2000;**39**(3):257-288

[90] Hoch FL. Cardiolipins and biomembrane function. Biochimica et Biophysica Acta. 1992;**1113**(1):71-133

[91] Houtkooper RH, Vaz FM. Cardiolipin, the heart of mitochondrial metabolism. Cellular and Molecular Life Sciences. 2008;**65**(16):2493-2506

[92] Klingenberg M. Cardiolipin and mitochondrial carriers. Biochimica et Biophysica Acta. 2009;**1788**(10):2048-2058

[93] Musatov A, Robinson NC. Susceptibility of mitochondrial electron-transport complexes to oxidative damage. Focus on cytochrome c oxidase. Free Radical Research. 2012;**46**(11):1313-1326

[94] Paradies G, Paradies V, De Benedictis V, Ruggiero FM, Petrosillo G. Functional role of cardiolipin in mitochondrial bioenergetics. Biochimica et Biophysica Acta. 2014;**1837**(4):408-417

[95] Schlame M, Ren M. The role of cardiolipin in the structural organization of mitochondrial membranes. Biochimica et Biophysica Acta. 2009;**1788**(10):2080-2083

[96] Nakamura K, Nemani VM, Azarbal F, Skibinski G, Levy JM, Egami K, et al. Direct membrane association drives mitochondrial fission by the Parkinson disease-associated protein alpha-synuclein. The Journal of Biological Chemistry. 2011;**286**(23):20710-20726

[97] Joshi AS, Thompson MN, Fei N, Huttemann M, Greenberg ML. Cardiolipin and mitochondrial phosphatidylethanolamine have overlapping functions in mitochondrial fusion in Saccharomyces cerevisiae. The Journal of Biological Chemistry. 2012;**287**(21):17589-17597

[98] Guo T, Gregg C, Boukh-Viner T, Kyryakov P, Goldberg A, Bourque S, et al. A signal from inside the peroxisome initiates its division by promoting the remodeling of the

peroxisomal membrane. The Journal of Cell Biology. 2007;**177**(2):289-303

[99] Monteiro-Cardoso VF, Oliveira MM, Melo T, Domingues MR, Moreira PI, Ferreiro E, et al. Cardiolipin profile changes are associated to the early synaptic mitochondrial dysfunction in Alzheimer's disease. Journal of Alzheimer's Disease: JAD. 2015;**43**(4):1375-1392

[100] The LipidWeb. 2017. Available from: http://www.lipidhome.co.uk/index.html

[101] Gao G, Wang Z, Lu L, Duan C, Wang X, Yang H. Morphological analysis of mitochondria for evaluating the toxicity of alpha-synuclein in transgenic mice and isolated preparations by atomic force microscopy. Biomedicine & Pharmacotherapy. 2017;**96**:1380-1388

[102] Taher J, Farr S, Adeli K. Central nervous system regulation of hepatic lipid and lipoprotein metabolism. Current Opinion in Lipidology. 2017;**28**(1):32-38

[103] Backman K, Joas E, Waern M, Ostling S, Guo X, Blennow K, et al. 37 years of body mass index and dementia: Effect modification by the APOE genotype: Observations from the prospective population study of women in Gothenburg, Sweden. Journal of Alzheimer's Disease: JAD. 2015;**48**(4):1119-1127

[104] Besser LM, Gill DP, Monsell SE, Brenowitz W, Meranus DH, Kukull W, et al. Body mass index, weight change, and clinical progression in mild cognitive impairment and Alzheimer disease. Alzheimer Disease and Associated Disorders. 2014;**28**(1):36-43

[105] Gerken T, Girard CA, Tung YC, Webby CJ, Saudek V, Hewitson KS, et al. The obesity-associated FTO gene encodes a 2-oxoglutarate-dependent nucleic acid demethylase. Science. 2007;**318**(5855):1469-1472

[106] Ferguson LR. Dissecting the nutrigenomics, diabetes, and gastrointestinal disease interface: From risk assessment to health intervention. OMICS. 2008;**12**(4):237-244

[107] Tau GZ, Peterson BS. Normal development of brain circuits. Neuropsychopharmacology. 2010; **35**(1):147-168

[108] NIH/NHLBI. Classification of Overweight and Obesity by BMI, Waist Circumference, and Associated Disease Risks. 2017. Available from: https://www.nhlbi.nih.gov/health/educational/lose_wt/BMI/bmi_dis.htm

[109] Barlett HL, Puhl SM, Hodgson JL, Buskirk ER. Fat-free mass in relation to stature: Ratios of fat-free mass to height in children, adults, and elderly subjects. The American Journal of Clinical Nutrition. 1991;**53**(5):1112-1116

[110] National Obesity Task Force. Clinical guidelines on the identification, evaluation, and treatment of overweight and obesity in adults-the evidenc report. Obesity Research. 1998;**6**:51S-209S

[111] Zhu S, Heshka S, Wang Z, Shen W, Allison DB, Ross R, et al. Combination of BMI and waist circumference for identifying cardiovascular risk factors in Whites. Obesity Research. 2004;**12**(4):633-645

[112] Third Report of the Expert Panel on Detection, Evaluation, and Treatment of High Blood Cholesterol in Adults (ATP III). National Heart, Lung, and Blood Institute. National Institutes of Health. National Cholesterol Education Program, 2001 May 2001. Report No.: 01-3670

[113] Lau WB, Ohashi K, Wang Y, Ogawa H, Murohara T, Ma XL, et al. Role of

adipokines in cardiovascular disease. Circulation Journal: Official Journal of the Japanese Circulation Society. 2017;**81**(7):920-928

[114] Ramos-Junior ES, Leite GA, Carmo-Silva CC, Taira TM, Neves KB, Colon DF, et al. Adipokine chemerin bridges metabolic dyslipidemia and alveolar bone loss in mice. Journal of Bone and Mineral Research. 2017;**32**(5):974-984

[115] Jung C, Fritzenwanger M, Fischer N, Figulla HR. Hepatocyte growth factor is elevated in obese adolescents. Journal of Pediatric Endocrinology & Metabolism. 2009;**22**(7):645-651

[116] Bell LN, Ward JL, Degawa-Yamauchi M, Bovenkerk JE, Jones R, Cacucci BM, et al. Adipose tissue production of hepatocyte growth factor contributes to elevated serum HGF in obesity. American Journal of Physiology Endocrinology and Metabolism. 2006;**291**(4):E843-E848

[117] Figlewicz DP, Woods SC. Adiposity signals and brain reward mechanisms. Trends in Pharmacological Sciences. 2000;**21**(7):235-236

[118] Wilding JP. Neuropeptides and appetite control. Diabetic Medicine. 2002;**19**(8):619-627

[119] Kurek Eken M, Sahin Ersoy G, Yayla Abide C, Sanverdi I, Devranoglu B, Kutlu T, et al. Association between circulating neuregulin 4 levels and metabolic, aterogenic, and AMH profile of polycystic ovary syndrome. Journal of Obstetrics and Gynaecology. 2019;**7**:1-6

[120] Comas F, Martinez C, Sabater M, Ortega F, Latorre J, Diaz-Saez F, et al. Neuregulin 4 is a novel marker of beige adipocyte precursor cells in human adipose tissue. Frontiers in Physiology. 2019;**10**:39

[121] Villarroya F, Cereijo R, Villarroya J, Giralt M. Brown adipose tissue as a secretory organ. Nature Reviews. Endocrinology. 2017;**13**(1):26-35

[122] Lee SA, Kallianpur A, Xiang YB, Wen W, Cai Q, Liu D, et al. Intra-individual variation of plasma adipokine levels and utility of single measurement of these biomarkers in population-based studies. Cancer Epidemiology, Biomarkers & Prevention. 2007;**16**(11):2464-2470

[123] Tan BK, Adya R, Randeva HS. Omentin: A novel link between inflammation, diabesity, and cardiovascular disease. Trends in Cardiovascular Medicine. 2010;**20**(5):143-148

[124] Supriya R, Yung BY, Yu AP, Lee PH, Lai CW, Cheng KK, et al. Adipokine profiling in adult women with central obesity and hypertension. Frontiers in Physiology. 2018;**9**:294

[125] Benchenane K, Berezowski V, Ali C, Fernandez-Monreal M, Lopez-Atalaya JP, Brillault J, et al. Tissue-type plasminogen activator crosses the intact blood-brain barrier by low-density lipoprotein receptor-related protein-mediated transcytosis. Circulation. 2005;**111**(17):2241-2249

[126] Korolczuk A, Beltowski J. Progranulin, a new adipokine at the crossroads of metabolic syndrome, diabetes, dyslipidemia and hypertension. Current Pharmaceutical Design. 2017;**23**(10):1533-1539

[127] Stofkova A. Resistin and visfatin: Regulators of insulin sensitivity, inflammation and immunity. Endocrine Regulations. 2010;**44**(1):25-36

[128] Rocha M, Banuls C, Bellod L, Rovira-Llopis S, Morillas C, Sola E, et al. Association of serum retinol binding protein 4 with atherogenic dyslipidemia in morbid obese patients. PLoS One. 2013;**8**(11):e78670

[129] Alkharfy KM, Al-Daghri NM, Vanhoutte PM, Krishnaswamy S, Xu A. Serum retinol-binding protein 4 as a marker for cardiovascular disease in women. PLoS One. 2012;7(10):e48612